# OPTIMIZING HEALTH FINANCING
## DIGITAL SOLUTIONS AGAINST HEALTH CARE INEFFICIENCIES, WASTE, ABUSE, AND FRAUD

JANUARY 2025

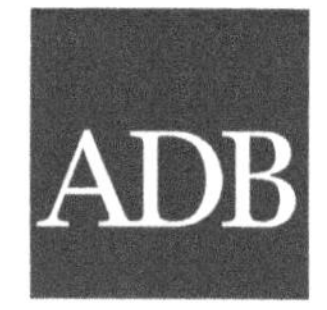

ASIAN DEVELOPMENT BANK

 Creative Commons Attribution 3.0 IGO license (CC BY 3.0 IGO)

© 2025 Asian Development Bank
6 ADB Avenue, Mandaluyong City, 1550 Metro Manila, Philippines
Tel +63 2 8632 4444; Fax +63 2 8636 2444
www.adb.org

Some rights reserved. Published in 2025.

ISBN 978-92-9277-168-3 (print); 978-92-9277-169-0 (PDF); 978-92-9277-170-6 (ebook)
Publication Stock No. TCS250024-2
DOI: http://dx.doi.org/10.22617/TCS250024-2

The views expressed in this publication are those of the authors and do not necessarily reflect the views and policies of the Asian Development Bank (ADB) or its Board of Governors or the governments they represent.

ADB does not guarantee the accuracy of the data included in this publication and accepts no responsibility for any consequence of their use. The mention of specific companies or products of manufacturers does not imply that they are endorsed or recommended by ADB in preference to others of a similar nature that are not mentioned.

By making any designation of or reference to a particular territory or geographic area in this document, ADB does not intend to make any judgments as to the legal or other status of any territory or area.

This publication is available under the Creative Commons Attribution 3.0 IGO license (CC BY 3.0 IGO) https://creativecommons.org/licenses/by/3.0/igo/. By using the content of this publication, you agree to be bound by the terms of this license. For attribution, translations, adaptations, and permissions, please read the provisions and terms of use at https://www.adb.org/terms-use#openaccess.

This CC license does not apply to non-ADB copyright materials in this publication. If the material is attributed to another source, please contact the copyright owner or publisher of that source for permission to reproduce it. ADB cannot be held liable for any claims that arise as a result of your use of the material.

Please contact pubsmarketing@adb.org if you have questions or comments with respect to content, or if you wish to obtain copyright permission for your intended use that does not fall within these terms, or for permission to use the ADB logo.

Corrigenda to ADB publications may be found at http://www.adb.org/publications/corrigenda.

Notes:
In this publication, "$" refers to United States dollars.
ADB recognizes "China" as the People's Republic of China.

Cover design by Josef Ilumin.

On the cover: Students are getting an education in front of computers at the Laguna State Polytechnic University in Los Baños, Laguna, Philippines (photo by ADB).

# CONTENTS

# TABLES, FIGURES, AND BOXES

# CASE STUDIES

# FOREWORD

In an era where universal health coverage is a global good that all countries must achieve, using digital technology to enhance the efficiency of national health financing systems has become essential. The Asian Development Bank technical assistance project *Using Digital Technology to Improve National Health Financing in Asia and the Pacific* has been supporting the comprehensive review and assessment of the status, challenges, and opportunities in implementing digital NHF systems across various developing member countries in the region.

The technical assistance project conducted detailed landscape analyses and country-specific assessments of the digital health tools and systems in seven developing member countries—Armenia, Bangladesh, Mongolia, the Philippines, Nepal, Palau, and Indonesia. The findings identified significant health service coverage and financial protection gaps, highlighting the need for robust digital solutions to accurately and efficiently capture and process health information.

The findings emphasized the importance of adopting digital health tools such as electronic claims submission and processing systems, digital clinical and health data analysis, and drug utilization review systems. These technologies are vital for transforming NHF management, ensuring quality of care, expanding access, and efficiently allocating resources.

Addressing fraud, waste, and abuse (FWA) remains a significant challenge in maintaining the efficiency and effectiveness of health care systems. This report explores the complexities of identifying and managing FWA within health systems, drawing on extensive quantitative and qualitative research conducted from April 2023 to March 2024.

The findings highlight the necessity of robust government actions, advanced analytics, and innovative technology to detect and manage FWA effectively. The report underscores the significance of various remuneration models and their impact on provider behavior, stressing the need for comprehensive systems to measure key financial and clinical indicators.

This report aims to guide and enhance national health financing systems through digital technology. Achieving universal health coverage involves complex processes, but with innovative solutions and collaborative efforts, progress can be made toward a healthier and more equitable future.

This report should be valuable in enhancing health system integrity and ensuring judicious use of resources. Mitigating FWA is challenging, but significant strides can be achieved with collective effort and innovative strategies.

**Eduardo P. Banzon**
Director for Health, Human Social Development Office
Sectors Group
Asian Development Bank

# ACKNOWLEDGMENTS

This report was authored by Thalia Georgiou, Asian Development Bank (ADB) consultant; Saro Tsaturyan, ADB consultant; Jae Kyoun Kim, health specialist; Akihito Watabe, health specialist; and Eduardo P. Banzon, director for Health, Human Social Development Office, Sectors Group, ADB, as part of ADB's regional technical assistance project, *The Digital Health Financing Support to Developing Member Countries in Asia and the Pacific*. The views expressed are based on quantitative and qualitative evidence gathered during the report preparation period from April 2023 to March 2024. Any recommendations or ideas presented are the opinions of the authors, and readers are advised to make decisions based on their judgment.

ADB employees and survey respondents from health care payer organizations across Asia and the Pacific assisted in producing this report. The authors would like to thank all those who generously provided their time and expertise in developing this report.

# ABBREVIATIONS

| | |
|---|---|
| ACG | Asia Care Group |
| ADB | Asian Development Bank |
| AI | artificial intelligence |
| CT | computed tomography |
| DMC | developing member country |
| DRG | diagnosis-related group |
| EHIF | Estonian Health Insurance Fund |
| FWA | fraud, waste, and abuse |
| GP | general practitioner |
| HIRA | Health Insurance Review and Assessment Service (Republic of Korea) |
| ICD | international classification of disease |
| KPI | key performance indicator |
| ML | machine learning |
| MRI | magnetic resonance imaging |
| NEP | National Efficient Price (Australia) |
| NHF | national health financing |
| NHI | national health insurance |
| NHIS | National Health Insurance Service (Republic of Korea) |
| P4P | pay-for-performance |
| TA | technical assistance |
| UHC | universal health coverage |
| WHO | World Health Organization |

# GLOSSARY

**ICD Coding.** ICD Coding is a medical coding system designed by the World Health Organization (WHO) to catalog health conditions by similar disease categories.

**Third-party administrators.** A third-party administrator is an organization that processes insurance claims or certain aspects of employee benefit plans for a separate entity.

**Diagnosis-related groups.** A type of case-based payment where a classification system used to categorize hospital cases into groups based on similar clinical characteristics and resource use.

# EXECUTIVE SUMMARY

## Background

Countries spanning Asia and the Pacific have made substantial progress toward realizing universal health coverage (UHC). Compared to a decade ago, millions of people now enjoy improved access to health care throughout the region. The coronavirus disease (COVID-19) pandemic was a stark reminder of how important this improved access is, with the relationship between health and economic prosperity brought sharply into focus. Despite this laudable progress, challenges remain. Population structures are changing; several countries are aging rapidly, altering the demand for health care and the population tax base to finance this. Noncommunicable diseases continue to be a challenge, with some markets seeing a near doubling of rates of diabetes and obesity compared with 20 years earlier. Climate change—once considered a challenge of the future—is already having a significant impact on health.

These challenges increase health care costs, pressuring public and private health financing schemes. Tough decisions are being made on benefit limits, co-payments, access models, and provision arrangements. However, health financing schemes are beginning to invest more heavily in technology, which brings big gains. Among these is the ability to run data analytics, which radically improves understanding of population health needs, how they are being met, how health care is being delivered, and what it costs. The insights from such analysis often deeply reveal inefficiency and ineffectiveness in health spending. The World Health Organization (WHO) estimated that 20%–40% of health expenditure is inefficiently spent, and improving spending efficiency to generate fiscal space has attracted substantial policy attention. Even a moderate improvement in addressing this issue may be the most effective way to sustain UHC.

The Asian Development Bank (ADB) implemented a technical assistance (TA) project *Using Digital Technology to Improve National Health Financing in Asia and the Pacific* in 2020. This TA aimed to support several developing member countries (DMCs) to assess their use of technology in health financing operations and support improvements through practical, strategic, and capacity-building initiatives. One of the key challenges observed and discussed with DMCs related to fraud, waste, and abuse (FWA) detection capabilities. While DMCs recognized FWA as a significant challenge, they were often unsure how to address these endemic issues. ADB commissioned a study to explore how FWA manifests in health systems, its challenges, and how technology can and has been used to leverage improvements. The study surveyed key stakeholders from public and private sector payers to gather views on the challenges and opportunities they see concerning FWA. The survey is understood to be the largest survey of its kind conducted in Asia and the Pacific and provides insight into the issues FWA creates in the pursuit of UHC.

## Key Methods

This report was compiled using qualitative and quantitative research methods. The study undertook a desktop review of document technologies and case studies that could offer valuable ways to address FWA. The study undertook a literature review to assess prior work in this field, though much of the literature on FWA focuses on the United States market. After assessing the relevance to the Asian context and identifying gaps in the literature in which primary research would likely add much to the overall analysis, the study surveyed health care payers across Asia and the Pacific. The appendix shows a breakdown of participant profiles of 239 respondents.

## Key Findings

The study identified several key findings that provided important insight into how FWA manifests in Asian health care payer schemes and how to address FWA. A summary of key findings includes:

- According to the survey, the most significant FWA issues were reported to result from provider behavior rather than member behavior. Commonly reported issues included induced demand, overprescribing, and the lack of consistent clinical pathways.

- Most health care payers surveyed did not collect key data in a structured form, which limited their ability to run basic FWA assessments. They also reported limited use of key performance indicators in their provider management approaches.

- Survey participants reported a low ability to challenge providers or members on issues related to potential FWA.

- Survey participants felt that many classes of technology would be useful for addressing FWA, but indicated that their introduction needed to be supported by appropriate system enablers such as data exchange standards and the consistent use of electronic health records.

- Many risk factors associated with FWA—such as lack of regulatory oversight of providers, unclear governance arrangements for FWA detection, and a lack of use of FWA detection tools—are common to many DMCs, making the likelihood of significant FWA high.

- The research indicated that structured data sits at the core of most FWA technologies, so an emphasis on achieving digitized claims would be a beneficial first step for payers to focus on.

- The research indicated that case studies on the successful use of FWA solutions are emerging from both advanced and emerging Asian economies, but these are generally not publicized widely, and more cross-country learning or cooperation could be beneficial.

## Key Actions for Governments and Health Care Payers

- Addressing FWA should be a policy priority given the considerable health financing likely lost to this issue.

- Investing in technology that supports health care payers in receiving claims data in structured forms is a vital first step in addressing FWA. This requires collaboration across the health system to ensure hospital electronic health records systems can "speak to" payer software, removing double entries and potential errors of providers. Data exchange standards need to be set by governments to ensure the integrity and safety of transmitted patient data.

- Implementing consistent use of international classification of disease coding would allow payers to appropriately analyze claims and undertake reliable local and international benchmarking to better detect FWA.

- Regulators and health care payers should consider collecting and publicizing data on key quality indicators, such as length of stay and readmission rates. This would help providers to see how they perform relative to peers and support improvement efforts.

- If payers use third-party administrators, responsibilities for detecting and preventing FWA must be clearly defined. Remuneration models need to be developed to reflect progress concerning FWA.

- Where possible, payers should consider using case rates or diagnosis-related groups to prevent oversupply and induced demand in provider settings. Investing in DRG software is likely to be highly cost-effective and support efficient claims management.

- Investing in professional fraud detection software—which can automate the identification of suspicious claims—is likely to yield positive results.

- Training and developing health care payer staff is a vital enabler of new models of working and successful technology deployment.

- Alongside technology investments, governance models need to evolve—including the requirement for registers of interest—to support potential conflicts of interest concerning policy and operational decision-making.

# WHAT IS FRAUD, WASTE, AND ABUSE, AND WHY IS IT IMPORTANT?

## Defining the Problem

In the complex interplay of modern health care systems, fraud, waste, and abuse (FWA) stand out as a formidable challenge, not only inflating costs but also undermining the integrity and efficacy of health services. This multifaceted issue affects all stakeholders—from health care payers and providers to patients and taxpayers—making it a critical area of focus for policymakers and health care administrators (Box 1).

Fraud involves deception to obtain financial gain unlawfully. These actions affect the health care system's credibility, from falsifying medical records to billing for services never rendered. The ramifications are far-reaching, as resources intended for genuine medical needs are diverted, leaving vulnerable patients without access to the care they require.

Waste—while not necessarily intentional—is detrimental. It manifests in inefficient practices, redundant procedures, and unnecessary tests or treatments and is perhaps the most widespread of the three issues. Wasteful use of resources inflates health care costs and exposes patients to unnecessary risks and discomfort. In an era where health care resources are strained, waste represents an opportunity for improvement and optimization.

Abuse involves exploiting the system for personal gain or convenience. This can take the form of overutilizing services, prescribing unnecessary medications, or subjecting patients to unnecessary procedures. The consequences of abuse are far-reaching, eroding public trust, compromising patient safety, and contributing to the escalating costs that burden individuals and society as a whole.

> **Box 1**
>
> ### Fraud, Waste, and Abuse Definitions
>
> **Fraud Definition:** Fraud in healthcare insurance involves intentional deception or misrepresentation made by an individual or entity, with the knowledge that the misrepresentation could result in some unauthorized benefit to the individual, the entity, or another party.
>
> **Examples:**
> - Billing for services not provided: Submitting claims for procedures, services, or supplies that were never provided.
> - Upcoding: Billing for more expensive services or procedures than were performed.
> - Kickbacks: Receiving payment or other benefits for referrals of patients or services covered by insurance.
> - Identity theft: Using another person's insurance information to receive medical services.

*continued on next page*

**Box 1** *continued*

**Waste Definition:** Waste refers to the overutilization of services or other practices that directly or indirectly result in unnecessary costs to the healthcare system. Unlike fraud, waste is generally not committed maliciously but through inefficiency or poor management.

**Examples:**
- Over-ordering tests: Conducting excessive diagnostic tests that are not medically necessary.
- Unnecessary treatments: Providing treatments that are not clinically indicated.
- Inefficient administrative processes: Redundant or inefficient administrative processes that add no value to patient care.
- Failure to coordinate care: Lack of coordination among healthcare providers, leading to duplicative or unnecessary services.

**Abuse Definition:** Abuse involves actions that may directly or indirectly result in unnecessary costs to the healthcare system. Unlike fraud, abuse does not necessarily involve intentional misrepresentation but includes practices inconsistent with sound fiscal, business, or medical practices.

**Examples:**
- Overcharging for services: Billing for services at a higher rate than is warranted.
- Misusing codes: Improper coding practices that result in higher reimbursement than appropriate.
- Providing unnecessary services: Delivering services that are not medically necessary or fail to meet professional standards.
- Failure to follow best practices: Not adhering to evidence-based practices or guidelines that ensure cost-effective care.

Source: Authors.

FWA in health care is not just a minor leakage of resources. Forensic assessments undertaken by governments and large health care payers have detected that 1.3%–10.0% was due to FWA (Table 1). It is a significant drain that costs billions of United States (US) dollars annually.[1] However, the survey on health care payers' perception suggested a higher percentage of total claims expenditures may have resulted from FWA (Figure 1). FWA represents a substantial burden on health systems, increasing the cost of health premiums and government subsidies and reducing the resources available for health care needs. The impact of FWA extends beyond financial losses. It undermines trust, compassion, and a commitment to patient well-being. When this foundation of trust and compassion is compromised, this will lead to delayed or denied treatments, compromised patient outcomes, and an erosion of public confidence in the health care system.

---

[1]    Taking even the lower of these estimates—applied to Asia and the Pacific's total health spending—would mean a figure in the billions.

### Table 1: Examples of Forensic Government Assessments of the Rates of Fraud, Waste, and Abuse

| Country/Region | Forensic Assessment Outcome |
| --- | --- |
| Australia | The Australian Institute of Health and Welfare estimated in a 2020 report that around $1.2 billion is lost annually to health care FWA, accounting for about 1.5% of total health expenditure.[a] |
| Canada | A 2019 report by the Canadian Institute for Health Information indicated that fraud and abuse could account for up to 5% of total health care spending, translating to billions of dollars annually across the provinces.[b] |
| European Union | Two studies suggest between 5%–30% of total health spending in the EU could be related to health care FWA.[c] |
| United Kingdom | The NHS Counter Fraud Authority reported in 2021 that the estimated losses to fraud in the NHS amounted to around £1.3 billion annually, corresponding to about 1.3% of the NHS budget. This figure includes fraud committed by both providers and patients.[d] |
| United States | A 2022 report from the Office of Inspector General of the US Department of Health and Human Services estimated that Medicare loses approximately $60 billion annually due to FWA, representing about 10% of the total Medicare spending.[e] |

EU = European Union; FWA = fraud, waste, and abuse; NHS = National Health Service; US = United States.

Sources:

[a] Government of Australia, Institute of Health and Welfare. 2020. *Health System Spending on Disease and Injury in Australia, 2020–21.*

[b] Government of Canada, Institute for Health Information. 2019. *National Health Expenditure Trends, 1975 to 2019.*

[c] European Healthcare Fraud and Corruption Network (EHFCN). *Study on Corruption in the Healthcare Sector. European Commission, October 2013.* Mossialos, E., et al. 2020. *Oxford Handbook of Comparative Health Law.* Oxford University Press.

[d] Government of the United Kingdom, NHS Counter Fraud Authority. 2022. *Annual Report and Accounts 2020–2021: Tackling Fraud in the NHS.*

[e] Government of the US, Office of Inspector General, US Department of Health and Human Services. 2022. *Semiannual Report to Congress, Fall 2022.*

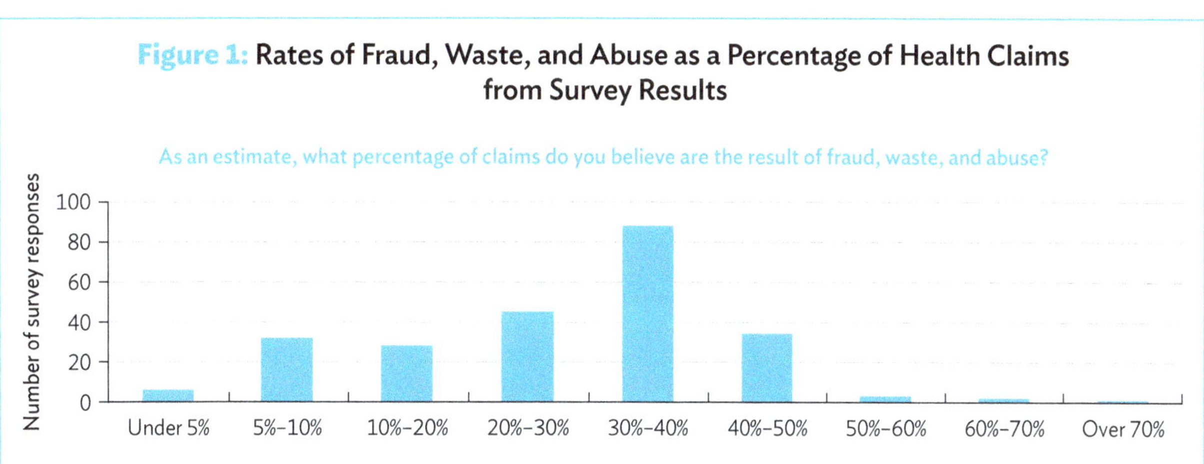

### Figure 1: Rates of Fraud, Waste, and Abuse as a Percentage of Health Claims from Survey Results



Notes: These figures are based on respondents' perceived fraud, waste, and abuse rates in their organization and/or the system more generally. This may be informed by respondents' review of their internal data; however, for confidentiality and improved response rate, the study asked this question based on perception.

Source: Survey of social and commercial health insurance leaders across Asia and the Pacific, conducted by the authors, 2023–2024. Total respondents size is 239.

# Addressing Fraud, Waste, and Abuse

Combating the pervasive threat of FWA requires a multifaceted approach involving robust regulatory frameworks, stringent oversight mechanisms, and an unwavering commitment to ethical practices. It necessitates a cultural shift within the health care system, where integrity and accountability are guiding principles that permeate every aspect of operations. It is imperative when addressing FWA to foster an environment of transparency and open communication where whistleblowers are protected and encouraged to come forward without fear of retaliation. The health care system benefits by empowering those in payer or provider environments to speak up against unhealthy practices.

Several factors contribute to the prevalence of FWA, with the lack of data analysis, limited provider management, and inadequate regulatory oversight being three of the most pervasive issues (Figure 2). The rapid development of health insurance schemes—often in countries where health care providers are fragmented and without national electronic health record standards—means payers often struggle to receive claims as structured data. This inhibits payers from utilizing the rich source of information claims data contains. Efforts are often placed on addressing claims costs claim-by-claim, which is time-consuming and often yields limited impact. In any health care system, there will always be exceptions—cases in which higher resource use or multiple claims for similar conditions—are justified. Payers' ability to address claims individually is, therefore, limited. Much more compelling conversations can be had when a payer can aggregate claims data and see patterns in how services are utilized, how care is delivered, and how this affects costs.

Quality indicators allow a comparison of institutions between and across regions. These indicators allow the documentation of clinical behavior during the provision of care, which can be used to improve and understand management processes and clinical pathways. Marked gains in the quality of clinical services have been observed in countries and systems that embrace robust transparency of meaningful quality indicators. Outliers are more easily identified, and practices and behaviors driving costs and care in unhealthy ways are much easier to spot.

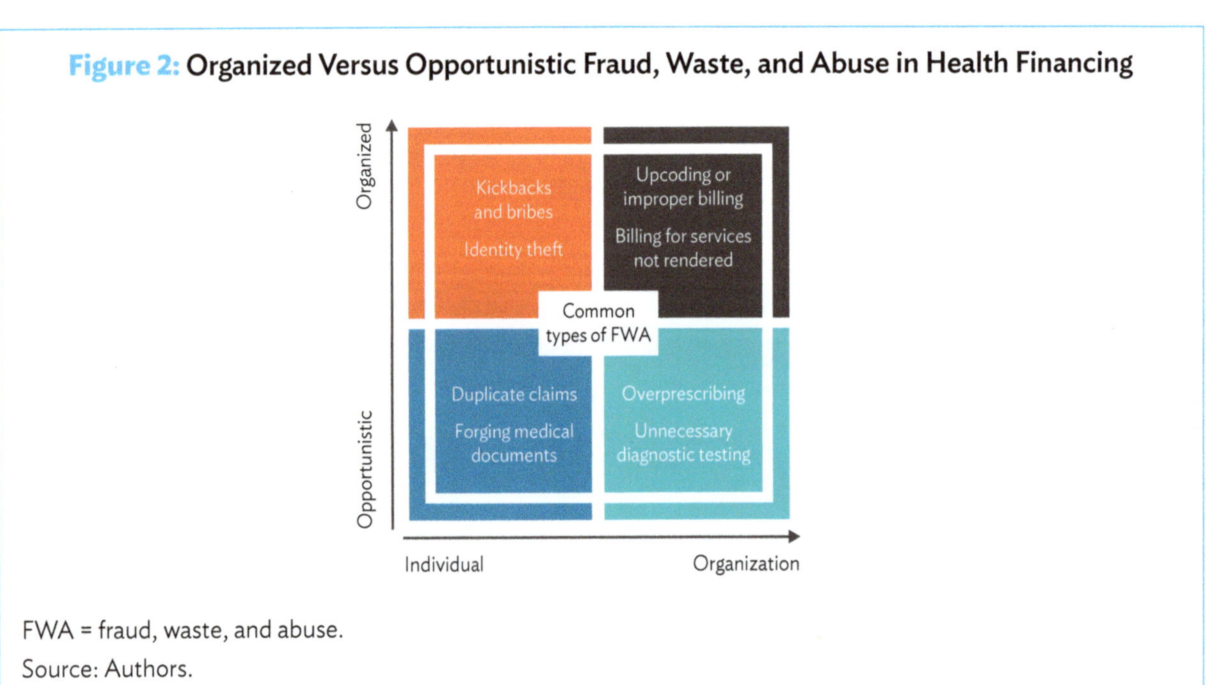

**Figure 2:** **Organized Versus Opportunistic Fraud, Waste, and Abuse in Health Financing**



FWA = fraud, waste, and abuse.
Source: Authors.

The approach taken by many health systems has historically focused on ensuring procedures and policies are in place within health provider entities, such as an infection control policy. However, providers often have little to no requirement to report the outcome of the care they deliver, making FWA harder to identify. This often means health care payers face impediments in accurately comparing quality and costs and inhibits providers from understanding how their services perform compared to peers.

While mitigating FWA is challenging, it has opportunities for innovation and improvement. As health care continues to evolve with advancements in technology and data science, the tools and strategies to fight FWA are becoming more sophisticated. Effective collaboration among governments, the private sector, and international bodies will be vital in creating resilient health care systems that can withstand the pressures of FWA. While FWA in health insurance presents significant challenges, addressing it effectively is crucial for safeguarding the integrity of health care systems and using resources efficiently and ethically to benefit all stakeholders. As innovation and collaboration continue, FWA can be significantly reduced, if not eliminated.

Addressing FWA is a financial endeavor and a moral imperative to uphold the health care system and ensure that every dollar and resource is channeled toward its intended purpose: preserving and promoting human health and well-being. It demands collective efforts of health care professionals, regulatory bodies, and the public to safeguard the integrity of the health care system and protect the well-being of those it serves.

# The Financial Impact of Fraud, Waste, and Abuse

FWA in health insurance can result in severe financial impacts in multiple ways. These practices escalate the operational costs of health financing providers and ripple through the health care system, affecting consumers, health care providers, and the overall economy. The financial impact of FWA on universal health care can be devastating. At its worst, it can undermine the scheme's sustainability and make the significant gains of many countries in Asia and the Pacific prone to failure. It is important to understand how financial impacts manifest and the challenges they cause. The research indicated that the financial impact of FWA has manifested in many ways, which collectively could erode payer viability.

## Escalating Health Care Costs

FWA contributes significantly to rising health care costs. The 2010 World Health Report *Health Financing: The Path to Universal Health Coverage* estimated that 20%–40% of spending on health was inefficiently spent. That figure could be conservative. The perception survey suggested that more claims might result from FWA. These costs arise from fraudulent claims for unrendered services, overbilling for provided services, and other activities that directly inflate the expense burden on payers.

## Increased Insurance Premiums and/or Government Subsidies

To offset the losses from FWA, health financing schemes often raise premiums. This makes health insurance more expensive for everyone, not just those directly involved in FWA. Higher premiums can have two profoundly detrimental effects. Optional schemes can lead to increased rates of uninsured individuals, as some opt out of purchasing insurance due to cost, thereby reducing the risk pool and potentially increasing premiums further in a detrimental cycle. In social or government-financed schemes with mandatory requirements to pay premiums—and governments subsidize those who cannot afford the premiums—the resulting higher premiums commonly result in more people needing to be subsidized by the government at a higher subsidy rate. All these options have consequences, presenting challenges for governments and the people served.

### Impact on Members' Benefits and Coverage

Payers may need to adjust the benefits structure to recover financial losses due to FWA. This could involve higher deductibles and co-pays, stricter limitations on coverage, and fewer covered services. Such measures can reduce the accessibility and affordability of care for many members, impacting their ability to receive timely and adequate medical treatment. In Asia, government and commercial schemes are moving toward more restrictive provider networks, often driven by cost.

### Resource Drain on Health Care Providers

Payers and health care providers bear the costs of combating FWA. Providers often need to invest in sophisticated compliance and auditing systems to monitor and prevent fraudulent activities, which can be costly. Additionally, the administrative burden of adhering to anti-fraud programs can divert resources away from patient care, affecting service quality. To ensure viability, health financing schemes that face high rates of FWA often begin to set fees that providers can charge, sometimes at unsustainably low levels, which can inhibit good providers from participating in schemes and limit their investment capabilities into new and better services. While limiting cost exposure, these blanket measures often fail to address endemic FWA.

### Government and Taxpayer Burden

Government-funded health programs are not immune to FWA; when these programs suffer financial losses, the burden often falls on taxpayers. The diversion of funds due to FWA means less money is available for other critical services or improving health care infrastructure, which can have long-term implications on public health outcomes. This is a particular issue in emerging markets, where resources are scarce, with competing demands for limited government funds.

### Reduction in Trust and System Integrity

The financial repercussions of FWA contribute to a general mistrust in the health care system. When members see their premiums rising and their coverage shrinking without a corresponding increase in the quality of care, their trust in the system erodes. This distrust can lead to decreased engagement with preventive care and hesitation to invest in health insurance, further destabilizing the insurance market.

### Economic Inefficiencies

FWA introduces significant inefficiencies into the health care system. Funds that could be used to enhance health care services or innovate new solutions are instead wasted on non-productive or fraudulent activities. This misallocation of resources affects the economic balance of health care and hinders growth and improvement in the sector.

## Clinical Impacts

The clinical impacts of FWA in health insurance extend far beyond the immediate financial ramifications, significantly affecting the quality of patient care and overall health outcomes (Figure 3).

### Reduced Access to Necessary Care

FWA often leads to higher insurance costs and premiums. As costs rise, insurance plans may become less affordable for many individuals, limiting their access to necessary health care services. Benefits might be curtailed to offset losses for those who remain insured, reducing access to essential treatments and services.

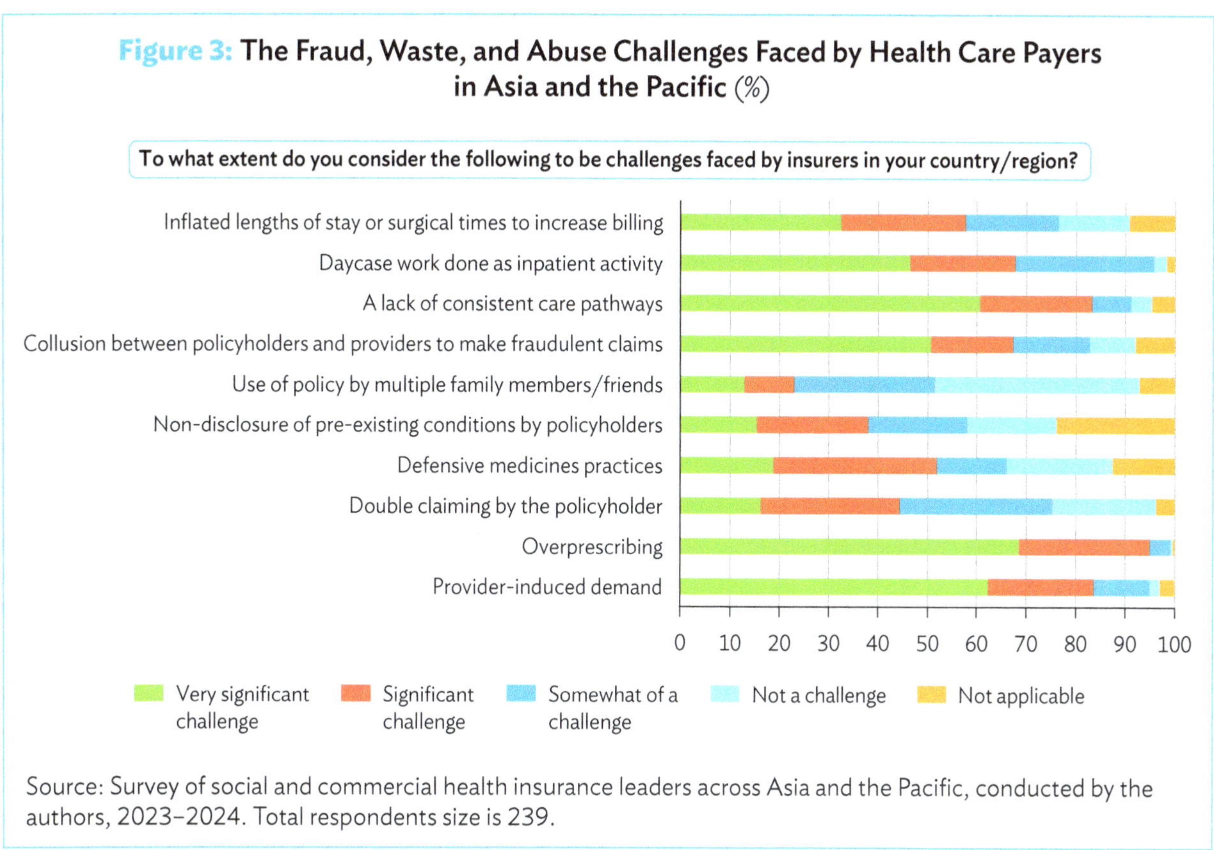



Source: Survey of social and commercial health insurance leaders across Asia and the Pacific, conducted by the authors, 2023–2024. Total respondents size is 239.

## Compromised Patient Safety and Care Quality

Fraudulent practices can directly endanger patient health. For example, billing for unnecessary procedures can expose patients to unwarranted medical risks from surgeries or tests they do not need. Conversely, in cases where providers under-deliver care to cut costs, patients may not receive the necessary treatments, leading to poor health outcomes. Instances of abuse where providers prescribe ineffective or inappropriate treatments can also jeopardize patient safety. Research indicated that many FWA challenges faced by health care payers in Asia and the Pacific are related to care delivery approaches, including a lack of consistent care pathways and provider-induced demand, which have real clinical implications for patients.

## Increased Patient Burden and Mistrust

Payers implementing stringent measures to counteract FWA can inadvertently affect genuine claims and services. Patients may experience delays in approving necessary treatments or encounter more significant bureaucratic hurdles. These obstacles can lead to dissatisfaction, reduced trust in health care providers and payers, and increased stress and confusion for patients navigating their care paths.

## Resource Misallocation

FWA diverts resources away from where they are most needed. The misallocation of funds and services inflates health care costs and means that valuable medical resources—like hospital beds, advanced medical equipment, and specialist time—may not be available for patients genuinely in need. In a stretched health care system, this misallocation can exacerbate wait times and reduce the overall efficiency of health care delivery.

## Erosion of Clinical Integrity

When fraud and abuse are prevalent, they can undermine the ethical foundations of the health care system. Providers involved in such practices might prioritize financial gain over patient welfare, eroding professional standards and ethics. This erosion can lead to a culture where such behavior becomes normalized, further deteriorating care quality and ethical standards in the medical profession.

## Public Health Risks

FWA in health insurance can lead to suboptimal public health outcomes. For instance, if fraudulent practices lead to widespread misuse of antibiotics, this could contribute to the development of antibiotic-resistant bacteria, posing a significant public health risk. Similarly, inappropriate medical practices driven by FWA can result in untreated conditions that become public health crises, such as the spread of infectious diseases that are not adequately addressed.

To mitigate these clinical impacts, it is crucial for all stakeholders—payers, health care providers, regulatory bodies, and patients—to collaborate closely. Improved surveillance, better regulatory frameworks, enhanced provider and patient education, and advanced analytics for detection can help minimize the prevalence of FWA and protect the integrity and effectiveness of health care delivery. Through these combined efforts, the health care system can focus more on providing high-quality, patient-centered care and improving clinical outcomes.

# MAJOR CHALLENGES OF ADDRESSING FRAUD, WASTE, AND ABUSE IN HEALTH INSURANCE

Health care payers face significant hurdles when attempting to manage FWA within their systems. These challenges stem from the complexity of health care transactions, the sophistication of fraudulent schemes, and the inherent limitations of preventive and detective controls. While offering many solutions for FWA, technology is simultaneously evolving novel schemes, so staying one step ahead will become a business necessity for health care payers.

## Complexity of Health Care Transactions

Health care billing and insurance claims are inherently complex and may involve multiple parties in some countries, as well as complicated services and procedural codes. This complexity can obscure inconsistencies and irregularities, making it difficult for payers to detect FWA. Each claim involves detailed information about procedures, diagnostics, and treatments that vary widely from one medical provider to another, adding complexity to the validation process.

## Sophistication of Fraudulent Schemes

Fraudulent activities in health insurance have become increasingly sophisticated, with perpetrators using advanced technologies and knowledge of billing systems to evade detection. Fraudsters often adapt quickly to new fraud prevention strategies. They employ complex schemes such as identity theft, provider impersonation, and elaborate conspiracies involving multiple fraud rings, which are difficult to unravel and prosecute.

## Data Volume and Quality

Payers deal with vast amounts of data, which can be positive and negative. While large datasets are necessary for advanced analytical techniques in fraud detection, they also pose challenges regarding data management, quality control, and timeliness. Poor data quality—inaccuracies, incompleteness, and inconsistencies—can significantly hinder the effectiveness of FWA detection systems (Figure 4). Moreover, integrating data from various sources often results in compatibility and standardization issues.

## Legal and Regulatory Challenges

Health care payers typically operate under strict regulatory environments to protect patient information and ensure fair claims handling. These regulations can limit the methods payers use to detect and investigate fraud. For example, stringent privacy laws might restrict access to or sharing of necessary data for effective FWA analysis. Additionally, varying regulations across different jurisdictions complicate the implementation of standardized anti-fraud measures or cross-border cooperation on health care FWA.

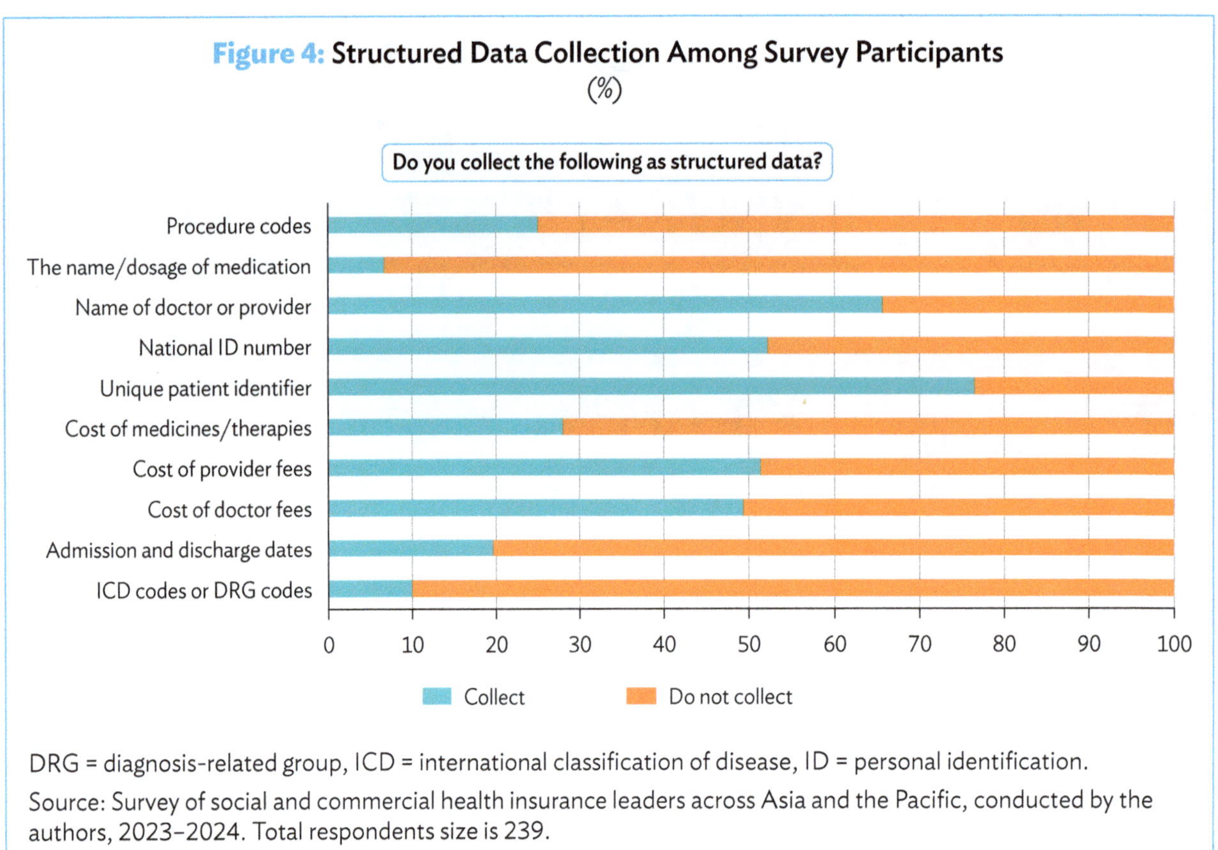



DRG = diagnosis-related group, ICD = international classification of disease, ID = personal identification.

Source: Survey of social and commercial health insurance leaders across Asia and the Pacific, conducted by the authors, 2023–2024. Total respondents size is 239.

## Resource Limitations

Effective FWA management requires significant investment in technology, personnel, and training. However, not all payers have the resources to deploy state-of-the-art systems or to hire and retain skilled professionals specialized in anti-fraud activities. Smaller payers may find these investments prohibitive, affecting their ability to combat FWA effectively. In these cases, health care payers often outsource some or all claims processing—including FWA identification and management—to a third-party administrator. In most cases, third-party administrators are not designed to address FWA and have very low recovery rates. They are often remunerated based on a percentage of the total claims cost, meaning there are often financial disincentives to addressing FWA.

## Detection and Prevention Technology Limitations

While technology is crucial for identifying and preventing FWA, it is not foolproof. The dynamic nature of fraud means that detection systems must continually evolve. Keeping up with the latest advancements in artificial intelligence (AI), machine learning, and data analytics is costly and technically demanding. Additionally, these systems can generate false positives that require significant manual review, straining resources further.

## Lack of Integrated Systems

Many health care payers operate on fragmented systems that do not communicate effectively with one another. This lack of integration can lead to gaps in the surveillance of transactions and impede the comprehensive analysis necessary for detecting sophisticated fraud schemes. For example, it is not uncommon for health care payers to have different systems for handling inpatient and outpatient claims or for claims systems to be fragmented between premium payment and underwriting systems. Health care payers often do not integrate with key health providers via, for example, an application programming interface. This often means claims are submitted in many forms, with PDF submissions still endemic across Asia and the Pacific.

## Cultural and Internal Challenges

Organizational culture and internal resistance can impact the effectiveness of FWA controls. Sometimes, the organization may have insufficient emphasis on compliance and ethics. In some markets, there may be inherent conflicts of interest, such as good friends or family working as providers and health care payers. Members may also have a financial interest in health providers, particularly the provision of private care, which limits the government's impetus to act. Anti-fraud measures may not be as effective without a solid commitment to combating FWA from all system levels.

By identifying and understanding these risk factors, health care organizations, and payers can develop more effective strategies to mitigate the occurrence of FWA, such as implementing stronger verification processes, enhancing data analytics capabilities, and promoting a culture of compliance and ethical practice (Table 2). As the landscape of health care and technology evolves, so must the strategies to protect the integrity of health insurance systems.

**Table 2: Common Risk Factors Facing Health Care Payers**

| Fraud | |
|---|---|
| **Inadequate Verification Processes** | Fraudulent claims can slip through without thorough verification of provider credentials, service delivery, and claim accuracy. This includes a lack of checks for duplicate claims or services never rendered. |
| **Sophisticated Schemes** | As technology evolves, so do the methods of committing fraud. Sophisticated schemes involving collusion between providers and patients, or even between different health care entities, can be challenging to detect without advanced analytic tools. |
| **High-Volume Billing** | Providers that consistently bill high volumes of services, especially those at high costs or high frequencies, may be doing so fraudulently, particularly if these services are not aligned with typical patient care patterns. |
| **Waste** | |
| **Lack of Clinical Training or Awareness** | Health care providers may order unnecessary tests or procedures out of an overabundance of caution or lack of awareness about the most current, evidence-based guidelines. |
| **Poor Resource Management** | Inefficient use of resources, such as medical supplies or pharmaceuticals, can lead to significant waste. This might include the expiration of drugs due to over-ordering or improper storage and handling. |

*continued on next page*

**Table 2** *continued*

| | |
|---|---|
| **Inefficient Health Care Processes** | Redundant or outdated processes within health care facilities can lead to unnecessary administrative or clinical steps that waste time and resources, contributing to higher health care costs without improving patient outcomes. |
| **Abuse** | |
| **Gray Areas in Billing** | Abuse often occurs in the gray areas of medical billing where the guidelines may not be apparent or are subject to interpretation. This includes misusing billing codes to receive higher reimbursements or billing for a covered service when a non-covered service was provided. |
| **Service Misrepresentation** | Providers may abuse the system by misrepresenting services provided, either to meet quotas set by administrative bodies or to take advantage of pay-for-performance measures. |
| **Manipulating Patient Encounters** | Some providers might schedule unnecessary follow-up visits or segment what could be one medical visit into several parts purely to increase billing. |
| **Common Contributors Across All Categories** | |
| **Technology Gaps** | Inadequate digital infrastructure and lack of integration across systems can create loopholes that fraudsters exploit. Poor data security can also lead to unauthorized access to sensitive information used in FWA. |
| **Regulatory Complexity** | The complexity of health care regulation and the insurance payment system can create confusion, which may be exploited to commit FWA. Complex reimbursement models and coding systems make it difficult for payers to detect inappropriate claims. |
| **Cultural Factors** | In some cases, organizational culture might inadvertently promote FWA, mainly if incentives align with volume rather than quality of care. This can also include a lack of emphasis on organizational compliance and ethics. |

FWA = fraud, waste, and abuse.
Source: Authors.

# THE USE OF TECHNOLOGY TO ADDRESS FRAUD, WASTE, AND ABUSE

## The Importance of Structured Data Collection in Managing Fraud, Waste, and Abuse

In the digital age—where data is as vital as currency—structured data stands out as a critical asset for health care payers. This type of data—which is systematically organized and easily searchable—offers numerous advantages that can transform how health care payers operate, innovate, and serve their customers. Ensuring structured data is collected is the most important first step in addressing FWA and lays the foundation for more advanced technologies to be implemented (Figure 5).

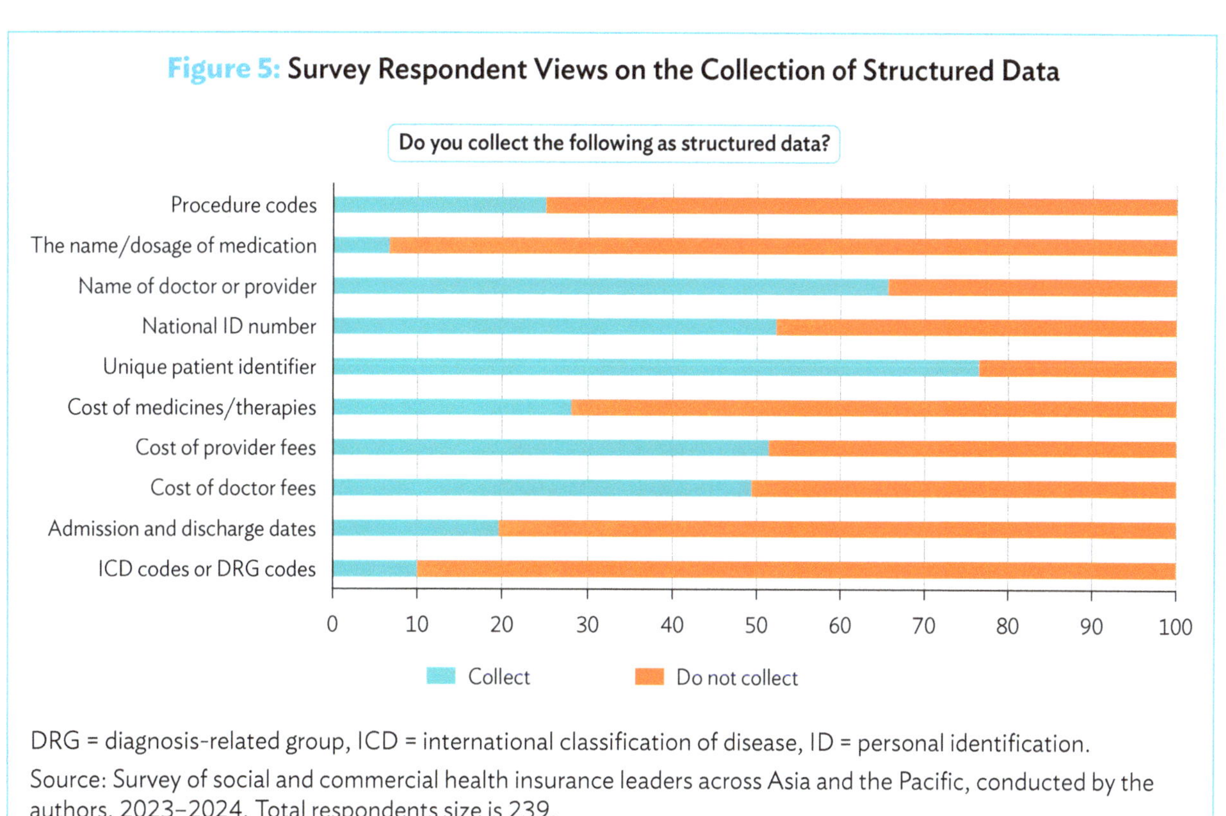

**Figure 5:** Survey Respondent Views on the Collection of Structured Data



DRG = diagnosis-related group, ICD = international classification of disease, ID = personal identification.

Source: Survey of social and commercial health insurance leaders across Asia and the Pacific, conducted by the authors, 2023–2024. Total respondents size is 239.

## Understanding Structured Data

Structured data refers to any data in a fixed field within a record or file. This includes data in relational databases and spreadsheets that can be easily entered, searched, and manipulated. Common examples of structured data in health care payer schemes include patient names, diagnosis codes, treatment codes, billing details, and other information that can be conveniently tabulated.

Structured data allows for the uniform collection and analysis of information, reducing errors associated with manual data entry and interpretation. This means improved accuracy in claims processing, member documentation, and compliance reporting for health care payers. Because structured data is aligned in rows and columns, it can be quickly processed with traditional database tools and algorithms. Health care payers benefit from this efficiency by handling large volumes of claims quickly and precisely, leading to faster response times, better ability to run FWA analysis, and improved member satisfaction.

Health care payers can make more informed decisions with access to clean, well-organized data. Structured data provides the foundation for predictive analytics, which payers use to forecast trends, identify risk factors, and develop new products that better meet the needs of their members. Structured data enables payers to segment their customer base effectively, understand population groups with unusual or high health care needs, identify providers performing well or poorly, and identify issues such as duplicate claims or patterns of potential FWA much more easily.

The survey results indicated that health care payer stakeholders from Asia and the Pacific understood the benefits of structured data. When asked about actions they felt the government could take to address FWA, the development of data standards, the enforcement of basic standards for electronic health records, and the use of unique identifiers all scored highly (Figure 6).

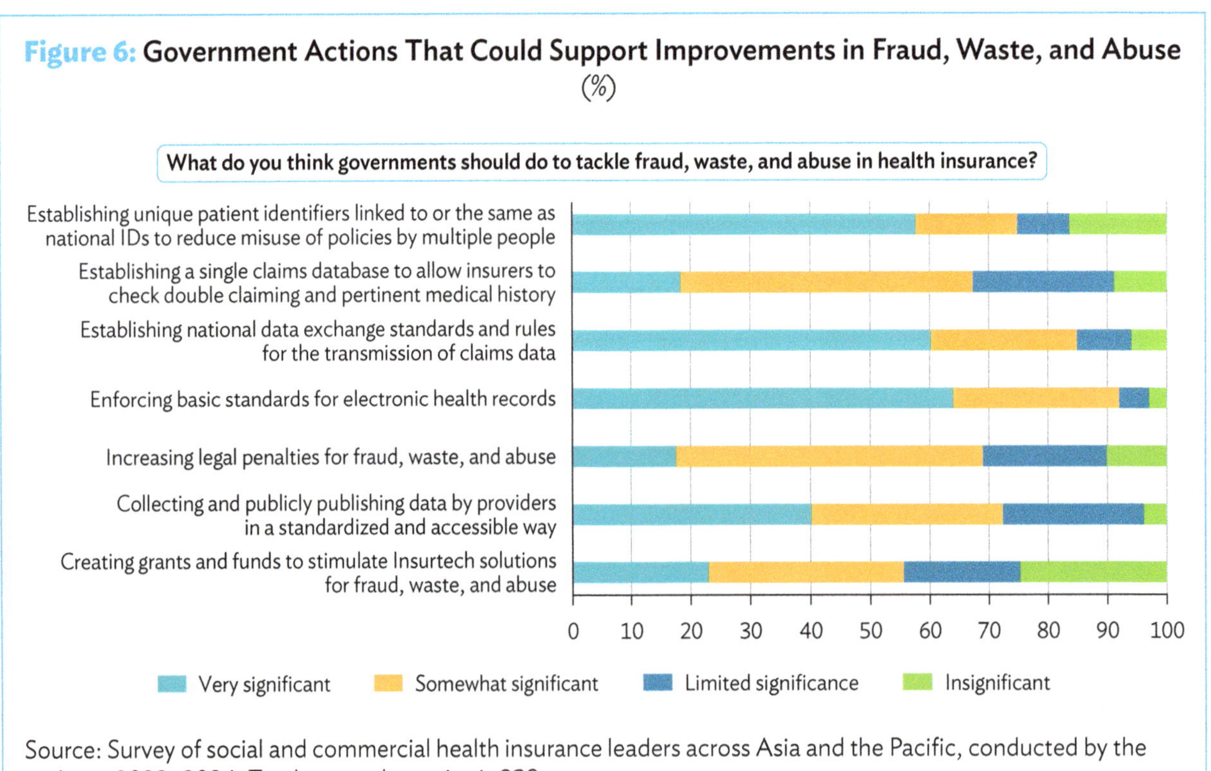

**Figure 6: Government Actions That Could Support Improvements in Fraud, Waste, and Abuse (%)**



Source: Survey of social and commercial health insurance leaders across Asia and the Pacific, conducted by the authors, 2023–2024. Total respondents size is 239.

While structured data brings many benefits, it also presents challenges. The primary concern is ensuring data quality and integrity, as even the best-structured system can falter if the data it contains is inaccurate or incomplete. As data privacy concerns continue, payers must also navigate the complexities of securely managing and storing personal and sensitive information. As technology continues to evolve, the role of structured data in health insurance will likely grow. Future advancements in data analytics and machine learning will further enhance structured data capabilities, making it an even more invaluable asset for payers aiming to optimize their operations and improve customer service.

# Leveraging Data Through New Technologies

As health care payers grow, the amount of data they manage also increases. Most health care payers understand that the sheer volume of data necessitates using systems that can scale effectively and support them in implementing the latest innovations in data analytics and FWA technology. Understanding these systems is integral to selecting tools that support operations and meet local needs and conditions.

In its broadest sense, technology is crucial for combating FWA in the health care system. Knowing where to start and how to ensure integration can be a challenge. This section assesses the most common technologies used for FWA and the benefits they could bring to health care payers. These technologies can help detect and prevent FWA and contribute to improving the efficiency of the health insurance system by automating routine tasks, ensuring compliance with regulations, and enhancing the customer experience by facilitating faster claim processing.

Most FWAs have at their core one or more forms of advanced analytics, which play a critical role in detecting and preventing FWA. These sophisticated tools and techniques can analyze vast amounts of data from various sources to identify patterns and anomalies indicative of fraudulent or suspicious activities. Table 3 describes the most common types of analytics.

**Table 3:** **Different Types of Analytics Used to Detect and Manage Fraud, Waste, and Abuse**

| Technology | Overview |
|---|---|
| **Predictive Analytics** | These tools use historical data to identify patterns that predict fraudulent behavior. By analyzing claims and other relevant data, predictive models can flag claims likely to be fraudulent based on similarities to past fraudulent claims. This can include anomalies in billing patterns, unusual treatment protocols, or claims from regions with high fraud rates. |
| **Machine Learning** | Machine learning models can continuously learn and adapt from new data, improving their ability to detect fraud over time. They can quickly process complex and large datasets, identifying new and emerging fraud patterns. For instance, unsupervised learning algorithms can detect outliers in data that do not fit any known pattern, which may indicate new types of fraud. |
| **Social Network Analysis** | This analysis examines relationships and networks among providers, patients, and claims to identify collusive fraud schemes. For example, if multiple claims originate from the same provider–patient network but show irregular treatment patterns or diagnostics, it may suggest organized fraud. |
| **Natural Language Processing** | These scrutinize unstructured data such as doctors' notes in medical claims or customer communication. Natural language processing can help identify discrepancies between what is written in text form and what is billed, revealing inconsistencies that suggest falsification or exaggeration. |

*continued on next page*

**Table 3** *continued*

| Technology | Overview |
|---|---|
| **Anomaly Detection** | Advanced analytics can set norms based on vast datasets and flag any deviation from these norms. The deviations are then investigated as potential fraud or abuse cases. Anomaly detection can be beneficial for identifying waste, such as overutilizing services that do not meet medical necessity criteria. |
| **Geospatial Analytics** | Analyzing data based on geographical patterns can help detect fraud hot spots or unusual patterns, such as many similar claims coming from an unlikely or unusual location. |
| **Real-Time Analytics** | This allows for the instant analysis of claims as they are submitted. Real-time detection can prevent the payment of fraudulent claims before funds are disbursed, enhancing the efficacy of anti-fraud measures. |

Source: Authors.

By leveraging these advanced analytical techniques, health insurance companies can significantly enhance their ability to detect and prevent FWA, saving costs and improving the integrity of health care transactions. This proactive approach helps stop fraudsters and deters potentially fraudulent activity by increasing the chances of detection and repercussions. Many respondents to the survey were exploring a wide range of technologies, though some—particularly more sophisticated technologies—were demonstrated to be at a much earlier stage of adoption (Figure 7).

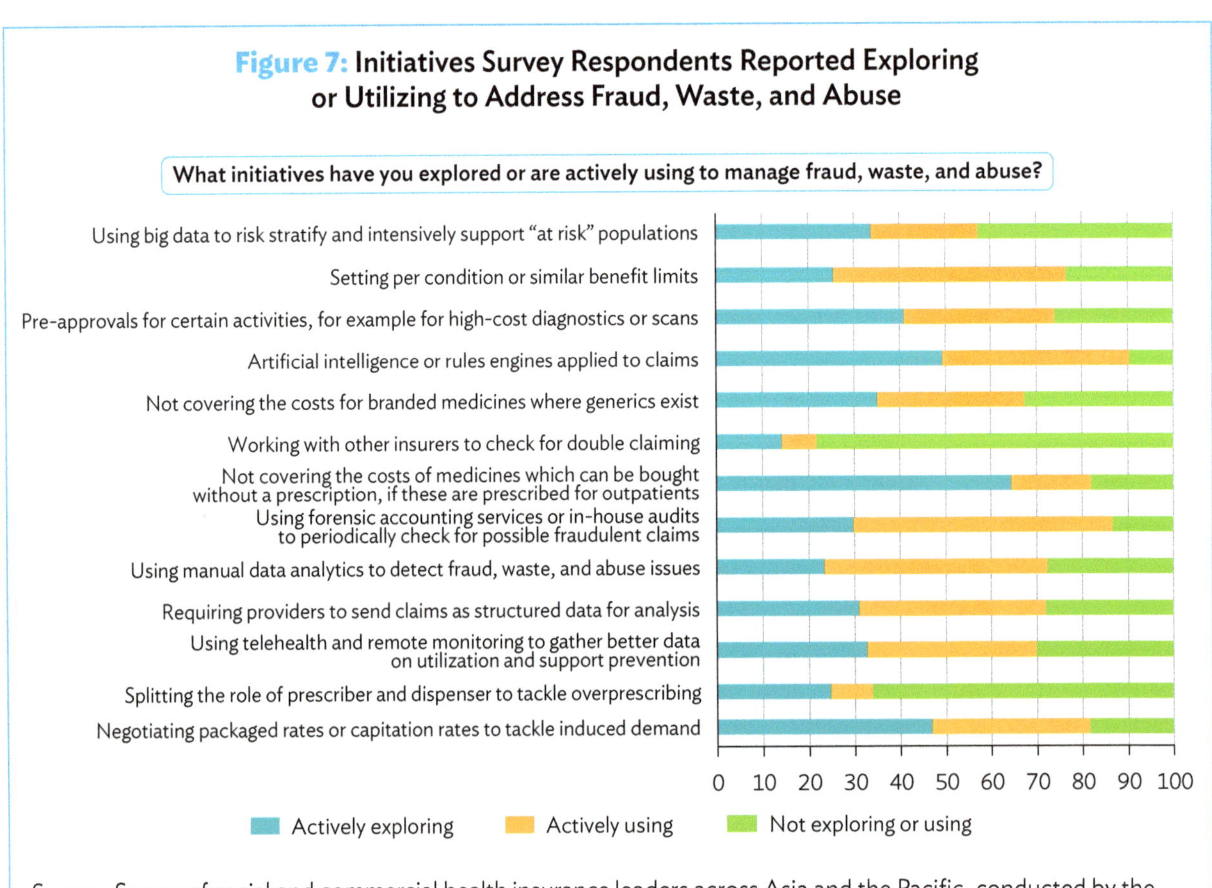



**Figure 7:** Initiatives Survey Respondents Reported Exploring or Utilizing to Address Fraud, Waste, and Abuse

Source: Survey of social and commercial health insurance leaders across Asia and the Pacific, conducted by the authors, 2023–2024. Total respondents size is 239.

## Case Study 1

# Shift Technology and a Tier 1 Health and Life Insurer

Shift Technology, a global leader in artificial intelligence (AI)-driven solutions for insurance, partnered with a major Tier 1 health and life insurer to address fraud, waste, and abuse (FWA) in their claims management process. The insurer, operating across multiple regions with millions of members, faced increasing challenges of detecting fraudulent claims using traditional rule-based systems. Shift Technology implemented its fraud detection solution, utilizing advanced analytics and machine learning to enhance the insurer's ability to identify and mitigate FWA effectively. The AI-driven platform was integrated into the insurer's claims workflow, analyzing data in real-time to identify suspicious activities. This included detecting patterns in claims data that might indicate fraudulent billing practices, provider collusion, or abuse of the system. Shift Technology's system was customized to align with the insurer's specific operational needs and regulatory requirements, making it both scalable and adaptable.

The partnership between Shift Technology and the Tier 1 health and life insurer delivered remarkable results, including a high detection accuracy with an 87% hit rate, ensuring that nearly 9 out of 10 flagged claims were confirmed as fraudulent or abusive. This accuracy allowed the insurer's Special Investigations Unit (SIU) to allocate resources more efficiently by prioritizing high-risk cases, thereby reducing investigation times and increasing operational productivity. Furthermore, the implementation of the AI-driven solution led to significant cost savings by preventing fraudulent payouts, enabling the insurer to redirect financial resources to enhance services for legitimate policyholders. In addition to fraud detection, the platform provided valuable data-driven insights that refined the insurer's claims processes and improved overall system integrity, all while scaling seamlessly to accommodate growing data volumes and expanded operations across multiple regions.

Source: Shift Technology. How We Helped a Tier 1 Insurer Detect and Prevent Fraud, Waste, and Abuse Cases. *Shift Technology Case Study* (accessed 17 November 2024).

Several important technologies back these analytic approaches. Blockchain technology offers a promising solution to the problems of data tampering and fraud in health insurance. By creating a decentralized and immutable ledger of all transactions, blockchain ensures that it cannot be altered retroactively once a record is made. This makes it extremely difficult for fraudsters to forge documents or tamper with transaction histories. Moreover, blockchain can enhance transparency in the billing process. Each transaction along the chain—from health care providers to payers and patients—can be tracked, making the process more transparent and accountable. This deters fraud and simplifies the claims process, reducing administrative costs and errors associated with manual processing.

Automated workflows and advanced case management systems can streamline the investigation process by automating data gathering, prioritizing alerts, and providing investigators with relevant context and evidence. This improves operational efficiency and enables faster resolution of high-value FWA cases. Biometrics, digital identities, and credential verification technologies can help ensure that only legitimate providers and patients are involved in health care transactions. This can prevent identity theft, impersonation, and other types of fraud perpetrated by bad actors (Table 4).

## Case Study 2

## Civica's Use of Fraud Detection Software in the Australian Health Care Market

Civica—a prominent software provider in Australia—has made significant strides in combating fraud, waste, and abuse in the health insurance sector. Their advanced analytics tools are designed explicitly for health funds and payers, enabling them to assess claims comprehensively for compliance and potential discrepancies. By integrating data from various sources, Civica's platform provides an holistic view of claims, allowing payers to identify patterns that may indicate fraudulent activities. This proactive approach enhances the accuracy of claims processing and streamlines operational efficiency. Health care payers utilizing Civica's solutions have reported impressive results, with some experiencing savings of about 10% in fraud-related losses annually. These savings translate into millions of dollars that can be redirected toward improving patient care and enhancing health care services. Implementing Civica's software exemplifies how innovative technology can play a pivotal role in safeguarding health financing and allocating resources effectively.

Sources: *Civica Fraud Solutions* (accessed 1 July 2024); Informa Insights. 2016. *Civica and Fraud Detection in the Private Health Insurance Industry*.

## Case Study 3

## Modum's Blockchain Technology and Its Impact on the Swiss Health System

Modum—a Swiss technology company—is revolutionizing the pharmaceutical supply chain through its innovative use of blockchain and Internet of things solutions, providing significant benefits for payers in the health care system. By ensuring the integrity and traceability of pharmaceutical products, Modum allows payers to verify the authenticity and compliance of medications throughout their journey from manufacturer to patient. This transparency is crucial for reducing the incidence of counterfeit drugs, which can lead to costly fraudulent claims and diminished trust in health care providers. With real-time data logging and immutable records on the blockchain, payers can confidently assess claims associated with medication use, ensuring that only legitimate products are reimbursed. This proactive approach minimizes financial losses related to fraud and enhances patient safety and treatment efficacy. Payers utilizing Modum's technology have the potential to see significant reductions in fraudulent claims, preserving their financial resources for more effective health care delivery and improving overall patient outcomes.

Source: P. Khedekar. 2023. Modum: Scaling Blockchain Solutions in the Pharmaceutical Industry. ResearchGate.

**Table 4: Technology Categories and Their Benefits to Fraud, Waste, and Abuse**

| | Technology Used | How It Helps |
|---|---|---|
| **Advanced Data Analytics** | • Machine Learning: Machine learning models are trained on historical claims data to identify patterns and anomalies. Techniques such as supervised learning are used to flag claims similar to previously identified fraudulent claims.<br>• Predictive Modeling: Utilizes algorithms to predict future occurrences of fraud based on trends and patterns detected in the data. This can include forecasting which claims or providers are most likely associated with fraud, waste, and abuse. | • Anomaly Detection: Automated systems scan millions of claims to find anomalies such as a high frequency of the same treatment from a single provider or unusually high costs compared to regional norms.<br>• Trend Analysis: Analyzing shifts in billing patterns over time to identify new or emerging schemes of abuse or waste. |
| **Natural Language Processing** | • Text Mining: Extracting meaningful information from text data such as clinical notes or billing information.<br>• Sentiment Analysis: Although more common in other industries, sentiment analysis can help assess the context within which medical notes are written, potentially identifying discrepancies in reported diagnoses. | • Fraudulent Claim Detection: Identifying discrepancies in the diagnosis and the treatment billed or spotting phantom billing through discrepancies in medical records.<br>• Compliance and Audit Trails: Automating the review of unstructured data within claims or patient records for compliance audits. |
| **Blockchain Technology** | • Decentralized Ledgers: Use of a decentralized database that allows multiple parties to hold a copy of the history of transactions, ensuring transparency and immutability.<br>• Smart Contracts: Contracts executed on the blockchain that automatically enforce and execute terms of agreement based on coded rules. | • Secure Data Sharing: Enhancing the security and integrity of data exchanges across health providers, payers, and pharmacies.<br>• Claim Adjudication: Automating the claims process with smart contracts ensures that claims are consistent with coverage terms and that payment is made only when all conditions are satisfied. |
| **Robotic Process Automation** | • Automated Bots: Software bots replicating manual processes, following rule-based logic to execute tasks.<br>• Integration Tools: Tools allowing robotic process automation bots to seamlessly interact with various data management systems. | • Process Efficiency: Speeding up claims processing by automating data entry and initial claim reviews, reducing the time and resources spent on these tasks.<br>• Compliance Checks: Automated systems ensure that claims meet all regulatory standards before processing, reducing the risk of accidental non-compliance. |
| **Social Network Analysis** | • Graph Theory: Utilizing algorithms based on graph theory to analyze and visualize relationships and interactions.<br>• Link Analysis: Techniques to examine and elucidate relationships and data flows between entities, such as providers and patients. | • Fraud Ring Detection: Identifying networks of providers and beneficiaries who exhibit unusual patterns of interaction that may suggest collusion or coordinated fraud.<br>• Behavioral Analysis: Understanding the relationship dynamics within data to identify influencers and key actors in fraudulent schemes. |

Source: Authors.

Deploying these integrated technologies can significantly enhance payers' ability to detect, prevent, and manage FWA across the health care ecosystem. However, it is crucial to have robust data governance, security measures, and experienced teams to leverage these solutions and adapt to evolving fraud tactics effectively.

---

**Box 2**

## Plan on a Page: A Quick Guide to the Basics Needed to Address Fraud, Waste, and Abuse

To begin running health insurance FWA assessments effectively, an organization needs to establish a robust technological foundation. The essential components of the base technology required are as follows:

### 1. Data Management System

- Data Warehousing: Consolidates data from various sources such as claims, patient records, provider details, and payment systems into a central repository, ensuring data integrity and accessibility.
- Data Quality Management: Ensures the accuracy, completeness, and consistency of data, which is crucial for effective analysis.

### 2. Analytics Tools

- Predictive Analytics: Uses statistical models and forecasting techniques to identify patterns that might indicate fraudulent activities. Machine learning models can learn from historical data and improve over time to detect anomalies more accurately.
- Data Mining: Tools that allow for the exploration of large datasets to discover patterns and relationships that might not be immediately apparent.

### 3. Reporting and Visualization Software

- Dashboard Tools: Provide real-time insights and visualizations to monitor key metrics and identify trends warranting further investigation.
- Reporting Systems: Facilitate regular and ad hoc reports to track FWA activities and compliance with regulations.

### 4. Fraud Detection Software

- Rule-Based Systems: Utilize specific rules or algorithms that automatically flag claims or patterns consistent with typical fraudulent activities.
- Anomaly Detection Systems: Identify outliers or exceptions in data that deviate from normal behavior.

### 5. Electronic Health Records System

- Integrates medical records across different health care providers to ensure that patient information is centralized and accessible, which is crucial for detecting duplications and inconsistencies in claims and treatment histories.

### 6. Security Infrastructure

- Data Encryption: Protects sensitive data at rest and in transit, ensuring that patient and provider information is secure from unauthorized access.
- Access Controls: Ensures that only authorized personnel can access sensitive data and systems, reducing the risk of internal fraud.

*continued on next page*

**Box 2** *continued*

### 7. Compliance and Audit Systems

- Automated Audits: Regular automated checks on transactions and claims to ensure they comply with coverage guidelines.
- Compliance Tracking: Tools to ensure all processes and transactions adhere to health insurance regulations and standards.
- Starting with these foundational technologies, health insurance organizations can effectively begin assessing and addressing issues of FWA to prepare for more advanced capabilities such as artificial intelligence and machine learning to further enhance their efforts.

### 8. Integration Capabilities

- Application programming interfaces: Allow for seamless integration between different software tools and systems, ensuring that the entire technological infrastructure communicates effectively and data silos are minimized.

**Implementation Considerations:** Implementing these technologies requires careful planning, including:

- Investment in Infrastructure: Substantial upfront investment may be needed to acquire and implement these technologies.
- Training and Development: Staff must be trained to use the system, interpret the data, and respond to potential fraud indicators.
- Change Management: Organizational changes may be necessary to support the effective use of new technologies.

FWA = fraud, waste, and abuse.
Source: Authors.

# Measuring Success: Important Metrics for Addressing Fraud, Waste, and Abuse

Health care payers need to monitor a range of key performance indicators (KPIs) to manage and mitigate risks associated with FWA effectively. These KPIs help assess the efficiency of detection, prevention, and recovery efforts related to FWA activities. They also help ensure that effective clinical services are being delivered and allow for more proactive provider management. Payers in Asia and the Pacific—public and private—have often been reticent to institute performance monitoring, fearing that it may mean providers leave their networks or raise concerns with governments. These fears have proved unfounded for health care payers who have remained. A clear set of measures removes ambiguity and often helps all parties understand what is expected and why.

One of the challenges health care payers face is unclear governance of their roles and responsibilities for performance monitoring within their organizations and the health system. The responsibility for ensuring care quality is often seen as a governmental responsibility. Countries in Asia and the Pacific are still establishing health care regulators that hold providers accountable. This vital responsibility is often neglected, which allows space for FWA to become more endemic. There is a significant need for health care

- payers to work with each other and the government to design the governance mechanism that will allow for efficient and effective care to emerge. Without regulation, health care payers must assume credentialing and provider management responsibilities to ensure financial sustainability and the delivery of high-quality care to members. Assuming this role will become a necessity rather than a choice.

The research indicated that most survey participants across Asia and the Pacific used some financial indicators—such as the total cost of claims—but few measured indicators associated with the quality or efficiency of health care (Figure 8). Indicators include the admissions rate for conditions that could and should be managed as outpatients or the rate of generics prescribed where such drugs exist. Quality metrics provide a rich source of information vital to managing FWA. Data on patient outcomes, adherence to clinical guidelines, and post-treatment recovery rates provide payers insight into how effectively health care is delivered. These metrics help payers identify top-performing providers and potentially develop preferred provider networks that promise better health outcomes and patient experiences. Such measures are vital in a health care landscape where value-based care is becoming more prevalent, shifting the focus from the quantity of services delivered to the quality of health outcomes.

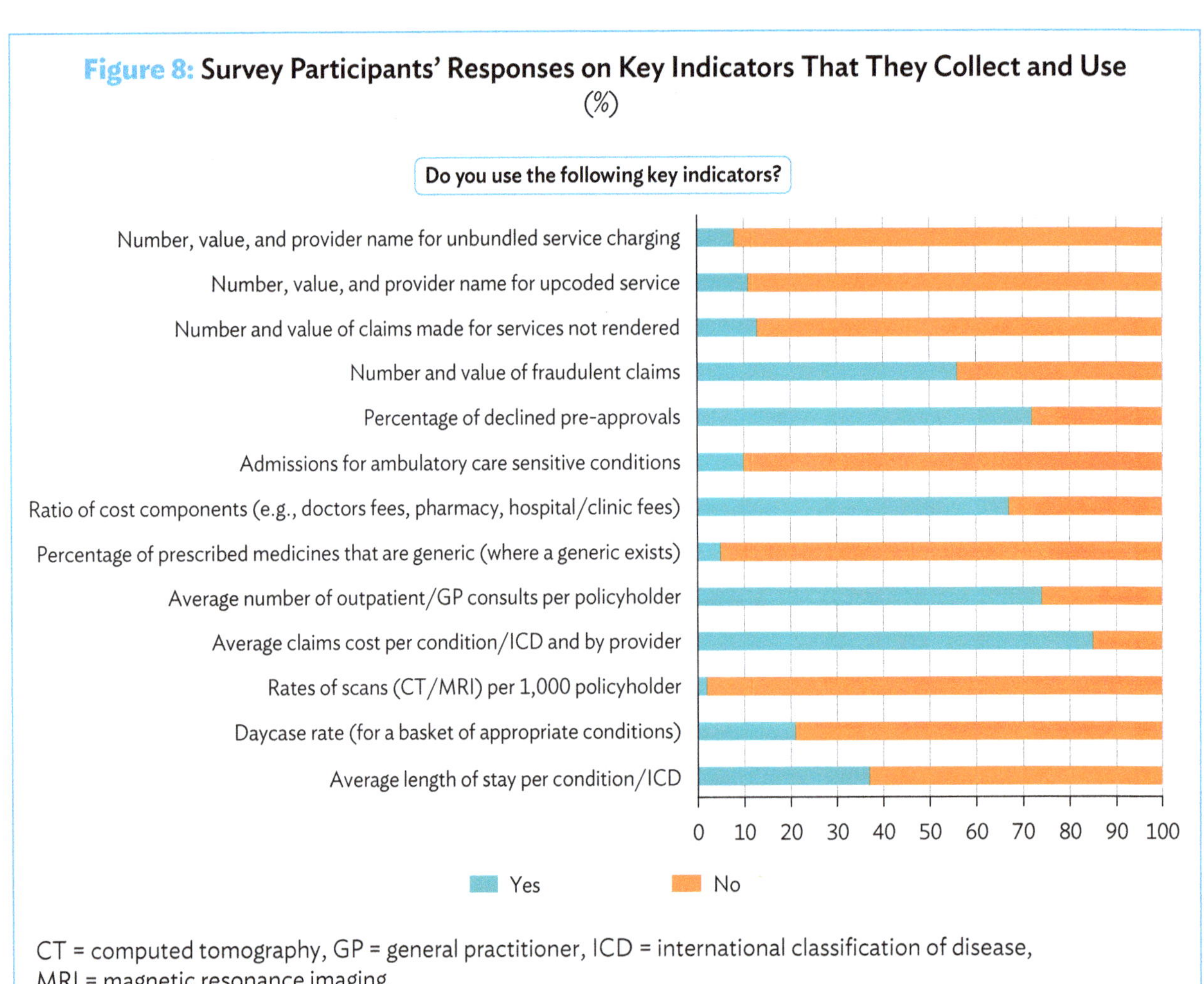



**Figure 8:** **Survey Participants' Responses on Key Indicators That They Collect and Use** (%)

CT = computed tomography, GP = general practitioner, ICD = international classification of disease, MRI = magnetic resonance imaging.

Source: Survey of social and commercial health insurance leaders across Asia and the Pacific, conducted by the authors, 2023–2024. Total respondents size is 239.

Monitoring provider KPIs also allows payers to manage costs more effectively. By analyzing data on service utilization, patient readmission rates, and complication rates, payers can identify trends that may suggest overuse of services or inefficient care delivery practices. This is crucial for controlling premiums and for ensuring sustainability in health care financing. For example, high readmission rates might indicate poor initial care quality or inadequate follow-up care, leading to increased costs for payers and patients (Table 5).

**Table 5:** **Key Financial Indicators Used to Measure Potential Fraud, Waste, and Abuse**

| Metric | Description |
| --- | --- |
| Fraud Detection Rate | Measures the percentage of claims investigated that are identified as fraudulent. This indicates the efficiency of the detection tools and methods of health financing schemes. |
| Fraud Prevention Savings | Estimates the amount of money saved through fraud prevention measures. This KPI helps understand the financial impact of preventive actions against potential fraud losses. |
| Amount Recovered | Tracks the total amount of money recovered from fraudulent claims. This is crucial for evaluating the effectiveness of the recovery process after fraud has been confirmed. |
| Average Time to Detect Fraud | Measures the time from claim submission to fraud detection. Faster detection can prevent further losses and is indicative of more effective monitoring systems. |
| Investigation Efficiency | Monitors the average time and resources required to resolve an investigation. This KPI helps assess the operational efficiency of the investigative team. |
| Cost of Fraud Investigation | Reflects the total costs incurred in investigating fraud cases, which provides insight into whether the investment in fraud management is yielding appropriate returns relative to the cost. |
| Claim Denial Rate for FWA | Indicates the percentage of claims denied based on suspicions of FWA. While a high rate suggests effective detection, it also implies overly stringent screening, negatively affecting customer satisfaction. |
| Change in the Incidence of FWA Over Time | Tracks the frequency of FWA cases over time to assess the long-term effectiveness of FWA management strategies. |
| Rate of FWA Referrals | Measures how often suspicious cases are referred for further investigation. A higher referral rate might indicate a more effective initial screening. |
| Impact of FWA Controls on Customer Satisfaction | Assesses how anti-fraud measures affect overall customer satisfaction. This is important because overly aggressive FWA controls might lead to dissatisfaction among legitimate claimants. |

FWA = fraud, waste, and abuse; KPI = key performance indicator.
Source: Authors.

Beyond measuring current performance, KPIs can drive innovation and improvement in health care services. By setting benchmarks and goals based on accurate and comprehensive data, payers can challenge health care providers to improve their services continuously. This can lead to adopting new technologies, treatment methods, and patient management strategies that enhance the efficiency and effectiveness of health care delivery. The monitoring of KPIs fosters transparency and accountability in health care.

When payers share these metrics with providers and patients, it encourages open dialogue about performance and areas for improvement. This builds trust between patients, providers, and payers and empowers patients to make informed decisions about their health care (Table 6).

**Table 6: Examples of Clinical Key Performance Indicators**

| Domain | Examples |
|---|---|
| **Quality of Care Metrics** | • Patient Satisfaction Scores: Measures patient feedback on their experiences and satisfaction with the health care provider.<br>• Health Outcomes: Assesses the effectiveness of care based on health outcomes, including improvement in patient condition, complication rates, and readmission rates. |
| **Utilization Rates** | • Service Utilization: Monitors the frequency of use of various services like emergency room visits, specialized procedures, and regular checkups to identify potential overuse or underuse of services.<br>• Prescription Rates: Tracks prescription practices, focusing on the appropriateness of prescriptions and potential over-prescription or under-prescription issues. |
| **Operational Efficiency Metrics** | • Measures the time patients wait for services, impacting patient satisfaction and overall efficiency.<br>• Tracks the availability of appointments, which reflects the provider's capacity and accessibility. |
| **Compliance Metrics** | • Adherence to Clinical Guidelines: Ensures the treatments align with accepted clinical guidelines and best practices.<br>• Accreditation Status: Keeps track of the provider's compliance with necessary health care regulations and standards. |
| **Patient Safety Metrics** | • Infection Rates: Monitors the rate of hospital-acquired infections, which is a critical indicator of the cleanliness and safety of the health care environment.<br>• Medication Errors: Tracks incidents of medication errors, which are important for assessing the safety practices in place. |

Source: Authors.

# Provider Remuneration and Fraud, Waste, and Abuse

Health care provider remuneration is a critical component of health care systems worldwide. It determines how health care providers are compensated for their services, influencing their behavior, the quality of care delivered, and overall health care costs. Various remuneration models exist, each with its unique risks and benefits. Each model has implications for FWA in health care. Understanding these dynamics is crucial for designing effective health care payment systems that minimize FWA while promoting high-quality, cost-effective care. Balancing incentives, ensuring proper oversight, and incorporating comprehensive performance metrics can help mitigate the risks associated with each remuneration model, fostering a more efficient and equitable health care system.

## Fee-for-Service

Fee-for-service is one of the most traditional forms of health care provider remuneration. Under this model, providers are paid for each service or procedure performed, including itemized billing for consumables and pharmaceuticals. This model incentivizes high care volumes, as providers receive more compensation by performing more services.

## Capitation

Capitation involves paying providers a set amount per patient per period, regardless of how many services the patient receives. Usually, the capitation model includes all consumables, pharmaceuticals, and other items required to deliver care. This model shifts some financial risk to the providers, incentivizing cost-effective care, but is typically used more frequently in publicly financed and delivered systems. Capitation can also encourage preventive care but may lead to underutilization and rationing.

## Pay-for-Performance

Pay-for-performance (P4P) systems compensate providers by meeting specific performance metrics such as patient outcomes, adherence to clinical guidelines, and patient satisfaction. There are few examples of full P4P schemes; many are a form of fee-for-service or capitation with performance-related positive or negative adjustments. P4P incentivizes high-quality care but may lead to metric manipulation.

## Case-Based Payments, Specifically Diagnosis-Related Groups

Case-based payments refer to a payment model where health care providers receive a fixed amount for treating a patient based on specific diagnoses or procedures rather than billing for individual services or procedures rendered. This model aims to control health care costs by promoting efficient care delivery and reducing unnecessary treatments, as providers are incentivized to manage resources effectively within the fixed payment framework. Diagnosis-related groups (DRGs) are a type of case-based payment where a classification system is used to categorize hospital cases into groups based on similar clinical characteristics and resource use. This system helps establish fixed payment rates for hospital services, incentivizing efficiency by encouraging hospitals to minimize costs while maintaining quality of care. DRGs are primarily used to streamline reimbursement processes and address issues related to oversupply (Table 7).

**Table 7: Remuneration Models and Their Relationship to Provider Behavior and Fraud, Waste, and Abuse**

| Remuneration Model | Benefits | Risks | Implications for Fraud, Waste, and Abuse |
|---|---|---|---|
| Fee-for-service (FFS) | 1. High Productivity: Providers are motivated to offer more services, potentially reducing patient wait times. <br> 2. Comprehensive Care: Providers may be more likely to offer a wide range of services, addressing multiple patient needs. | 1. Overutilization: The primary risk of FFS is the potential for overutilization of services, as providers might perform unnecessary procedures to increase revenue. <br> 2. Quality of Care: The focus on quantity over quality can lead to suboptimal patient outcomes, with providers prioritizing volume over the efficacy of treatments. | FFS systems are particularly susceptible to FWA. Providers may engage in upcoding, billing for more expensive services than those provided, or performing unnecessary procedures to maximize payments, leading to significant financial losses for health care systems. |

*continued on next page*

**Table 7** *continued*

| Remuneration Model | Benefits | Risks | Implications for Fraud, Waste, and Abuse |
|---|---|---|---|
| Capitation | 1. Cost Control: By providing a fixed payment, capitation encourages providers to manage resources efficiently and avoid unnecessary services.<br>2. Preventive Care: Providers are financially incentivized to keep patients healthy, as healthier patients require fewer costly interventions. | 1. Underutilization: There is a risk that providers might skimp on necessary care to save costs, potentially leading to poor patient outcomes.<br>2. Provider Burden: Providers bear the financial risk if patient care costs exceed the capitation payment, which can be particularly challenging with high-need patients. | Capitation reduces opportunities for fraud common in FFS, such as billing for unnecessary services. However, it can lead to underutilization fraud, where providers might avoid necessary but costly treatments. Ensuring quality care and proper oversight is crucial to mitigate these risks. |
| Pay-for-performance (P4P) | 1. Improved Quality: P4P encourages providers to focus on delivering high-quality care by tying compensation to performance.<br>2. Patient Satisfaction: Providers are incentivized to improve patient experiences and outcomes, potentially increasing patient satisfaction. | 1. Metric Manipulation: Providers might focus on meeting specific metrics at the expense of other aspects of care, potentially leading to gaming the system.<br>2. Unequal Impact: Providers serving high-risk or socioeconomically disadvantaged populations might face financial penalties and struggle to meet performance metrics. | P4P aims to reduce waste by rewarding effective care. However, it can lead to new forms of abuse such as manipulating patient records to meet performance targets or focusing on easily achievable metrics while neglecting broader aspects of care. |
| Diagnosis-related groups (DRGs) | 1. Cost control: DRGs help set predetermined procedure rates, allowing payers to control costs by offering fixed reimbursements regardless of actual resources used.<br>2. Predictability: DRGs provide financial predictability, making it easier for payers to budget and forecast expenses.<br>3. Efficiency incentives: Hospitals are incentivized to be more efficient, as they will only receive a set amount per patient case, encouraging shorter stays and resource management. | 1. Inaccurate classification: If a patient's condition is miscoded into a higher DRG, payers might overpay for services, leading to potential losses.<br>2. Undertreatment risk: To stay within the fixed reimbursement, hospitals might cut costs, leading to undertreatment of patients.<br>3. Variability in care complexity: DRGs may not fully account for the complexity of some instances, leaving payers vulnerable to cost increases for outlier patients. | DRGs are generally regarded as ways to incentivize efficiency. However, there are several risks. These include upcoding by which providers might fraudulently assign higher-paying DRGs to increase reimbursement. There may also be an incentive to admit patients unnecessarily or prolong hospital stays to maximize reimbursement within the DRG framework. |

FWA = fraud, waste, and abuse.

Source: Authors.

Case Study 4

## The Adoption of 3M's Diagnosis-Related Group Software and Its Impact on Fraud, Waste, and Abuse

3M Health Information Systems has been at the forefront of transforming health care billing and coding practices through its advanced diagnosis-related group software, which is widely utilized by hospitals and payers in the United States and internationally. This innovative technology streamlines the classification of diagnoses and treatments, ensuring that health care providers accurately code patient encounters according to established standards. By automating the coding process and integrating robust analytics, 3M's system helps identify discrepancies and potential errors in billing before claims are submitted. This proactive approach minimizes the risk of denials and audits and fosters improved provider behaviors by emphasizing accuracy and compliance. As a result, health care organizations leveraging 3M's diagnosis-related group software have reported significant reductions in billing errors, leading to an estimated savings of up to 20% in denied claims and fraudulent billing. These cost savings enhance financial stability for providers, allowing them to focus more on delivering high-quality patient care rather than navigating complex billing disputes. The deployment of 3M's technology illustrates the powerful impact that sophisticated coding solutions can have on improving operational efficiency and promoting integrity within the health care financing system.

Source: 3M Health Information Systems (accessed September 2024).

Case Study 5

## Japan's Capitation Model in Elder Care

Japan introduced its long-term care insurance system in 2000 to address its rapidly aging population. A key feature of this system is the capitation model, which reimburses health care providers a fixed amount per enrolled patient over a specified period, regardless of the services used. This model combines with a fee-for-service structure that incentivizes providers to manage care efficiently while maintaining care quality. Under this system, the payment structure includes a basic capitation fee and additional payments for more complex or resource-intensive cases.

### Benefits of Capitation

(i) **Cost Control and Predictability:** Capitation enables Japan's health care system to manage costs effectively. By allocating a fixed amount per patient, health care providers have a clear budget for managing long-term care, which helps control overall expenditure. It also allows for more predictable health care budgets, which is vital for Japan given its high percentage of elderly citizens (28.1% aged 65 or older in 2018).

*continued on next page*

**Case Study 5** *continued*

(ii) **Encourages Preventive Care:** Since providers receive a fixed payment, they are incentivized to focus on preventive measures to keep elderly patients healthier and reduce the likelihood of expensive, resource-intensive treatments. This aligns with Japan's focus on reducing the progression of care needs, as highlighted in the regular revisions to the long-term care insurance payment system.

(iii) **Integrated Care Approach:** The capitation model in Japan fosters the development of community-based integrated care systems. These systems encourage collaboration between various care providers, such as hospitals, rehabilitation centers, and home care services, creating a more holistic approach to elder care. This integration helps streamline patient management and ensures better coordination of care.

## Risks and Challenges

(i) **Risk of Undertreatment:** One of the main concerns with capitation is that it may lead to undertreatment. Providers may minimize their services to stay within the fixed capitation payment. This could result in lower-quality care for elderly patients, particularly those with complex or rapidly changing health conditions.

(ii) **Increased Administrative Burden:** Monitoring and adjusting payments to ensure they match the care needs of patients can be complex. Providers must document patient care thoroughly, and regular reassessments are necessary to prevent underfunding for those with more severe conditions. This results in an increased administrative load on care providers and government bodies.

(iii) **Incentive for Selective Enrollment:** Providers may be incentivized to avoid enrolling patients with severe or chronic conditions requiring more intensive care, as these patients could strain the fixed capitation budgets. This could lead to inequitable access to care, particularly for those with the highest needs.

Japan's capitation model has allowed for more predictable health care costs and encouraged preventive care, essential in managing a rapidly aging population. However, the model also presents risks, particularly regarding potential undertreatment and the administrative complexity required to balance patient needs and resources. Continuous monitoring and adjustments to the system are necessary to ensure that the benefits of capitation outweigh its risks.

Sources: N. Tamiya et al. 2020. Outcomes of Long-term Care Insurance Services in Japan: Evidence from National Long-term Care Insurance Claim Data. Economic Research Institute for ASEAN and East Asia Research Project Report; Government of Japan, Ministry of Health, Labour and Welfare. 2020. Long-term Care Insurance System in Japan.

Case Study 6

# Fee-for-Service in Public Hospitals in the People's Republic of China

The health care system in the People's Republic of China (PRC)—particularly in public hospitals—predominantly operates under a fee-for-service (FFS) model. This model means hospitals and health care providers are compensated based on the number and type of services rendered. Each procedure, diagnostic test, or treatment is billed separately, and providers are reimbursed. Public hospitals comprise the backbone of health care services in the PRC, providing over 90% of inpatient services.

The FFS model in the PRC developed as a means to incentivize health care providers during the economic reforms of the 1980s when public hospitals had to generate income. The model allowed public hospitals to charge patients for services beyond basic care, driving up service offerings and modernizing care delivery.

## Benefits of the Fee-for-Service Model

(i)   **Incentive for Increased Service Provision:** The FFS model encourages hospitals and physicians to provide a wide range of services, from advanced diagnostics to complex surgeries. This can lead to more comprehensive patient care, financially incentivizing physicians to offer thorough diagnostics and treatments.

(ii)  **Revenue Generation for Hospitals:** The government partially funds public hospitals in the PRC but relies significantly on service fees to sustain operations. The FFS model provides an essential revenue stream for hospitals, allowing them to invest in modern equipment, advanced treatments, and medical staff.

(iii) **Encourages Specialization:** Hospitals and physicians are encouraged to develop specialized services and offer cutting-edge treatments to attract more patients. This dynamic fosters the growth of medical expertise and advances in certain areas of health care, particularly in urban hospitals.

## Risks and Challenges of the Fee-for-Service Model

(i)   **Over-treatment and Over-Medicalization:** One of the key risks associated with FFS is the tendency for over-treatment. Since providers are paid for every service, there is a financial incentive to order unnecessary tests, prescribe more medications, or perform additional procedures. This can lead to higher patient costs and potentially expose them to unnecessary medical risks.

(ii)  **Cost Burden on Patients:** The FFS model can burden patients financially, particularly those requiring long-term or chronic care. Even with public insurance programs in place, out-of-pocket expenses for patients can be significant, especially for services that fall outside basic coverage.

(iii) **Focus on Profit-Driven Care:** The FFS system encourages hospitals to focus on high-revenue procedures and services, sometimes at the expense of basic or preventive care. This can lead to a health care environment where treatments that generate more income are prioritized, while essential but less profitable care, such as routine check-ups or public health initiatives, may receive less attention.

*continued on next page*

**Case Study 6** *continued*

**Implications for Fraud, Waste, and Abuse**

(i) **Overuse of Diagnostics and Pharmaceuticals:** There is a documented trend of overuse of diagnostic tests, medications, and procedures in the Chinese health care system. Physicians may prescribe unnecessary treatments to increase their revenue under the FFS model. For example, excessive use of intravenous drips—which is common in the PRC—is often driven by financial incentives rather than clinical necessity.

(ii) **Health Care Inequity:** The FFS model exacerbates inequalities in access to care, particularly between urban and rural regions. Urban hospitals—which can offer more services—attract wealthier patients, while rural hospitals often struggle to generate revenue due to lower patient volumes and fewer advanced services.

The PRC FFS model in public hospitals has facilitated the modernization and expansion of health care services, driving revenue and incentivizing comprehensive care. However, it also presents significant risks, particularly in over-treatment, increased patient costs, and the prioritization of profit-driven services. As the PRC moves toward health care reforms, balancing the benefits of service expansion with the risks of overuse and inequity remains a key challenge.

Sources: World Health Organization. 2015. People's Republic of China Health System Review. *Health Systems in Transition.* 5 (7); Q. Meng, et al. 2019. China's Health System Reforms: Review of 10 Years of Progress. BMJ; M. Liu, et al. 2021. Effects of Chinese Medical Pricing Reform on the Structure of Hospital Revenue and Healthcare Expenditure in County Hospital: An Interrupted Time Series Analysis. *BMC Health Serv Res.* 21 (1).

# LESSONS FROM AROUND THE GLOBE: SUCCESSFUL EFFORTS TO ADDRESS FRAUD, WASTE, AND ABUSE

## Learning from Global Experience

Globally, health care payers are beginning to address FWA through various technological approaches. These early case studies provide valuable insights into the possibilities and challenges of integrating technology into health care payer systems. These efforts highlight the importance of continuous innovation and adaptation in the face of evolving threats and technological advancements. This section explores some of these case studies, emphasizing the technology employed and the outcomes achieved. Common across all are the success factors, which include careful integration with existing systems, thorough training for staff, and strong data security measures. The challenges primarily revolve around the initial cost and complexity of implementing sophisticated AI systems and the ongoing need for updates and maintenance to keep the systems effective against new fraud tactics.

### Case Study 7

### The Development of Estonia's e-Health Systems and Their Impact on Fraud, Waste, and Abuse

#### Overview

Estonia has been at the forefront of digital transformation in health care, employing advanced technologies to streamline operations and improve efficiency. One key area of focus has been reducing fraud, waste, and abuse (FWA) in health care claims processing. Through integrating a digital invoicing system and machine learning (ML), Estonia's health care system—particularly through the Estonian Health Insurance Fund (EHIF)—has improved its ability to monitor claims, detect fraudulent activity, and enhance service delivery.

#### Problem

Despite Estonia's position as an early adopter of e-health solutions, its claims processing system struggled with inefficiencies, administrative burdens, and inaccuracies. These issues created vulnerabilities in the system, where FWA could go undetected due to a lack of robust verification methods. Delays in claims processing also resulted in longer patient wait times and slower reimbursements for health care providers, further straining the system.

*continued on next page*

**Case Study 7** *continued*

## Solution: Digital Invoicing and Machine Learning

To address these challenges, Estonia implemented a digital invoicing system integrating automated controls to verify real-time claims. Integrating ML models within this system has greatly improved the accuracy and speed of fraud detection while reducing the manual workload required for claims processing. The system had some of the following features and benefits:

(i)   **Automated Claims Verification:** The digital invoicing system employs 368 automated controls to review claims before processing payments. These controls ensure all claims adhere to predefined guidelines, minimizing errors and inconsistencies.

(ii)  **Machine Learning for Fraud Detection:** ML algorithms—supervised and unsupervised—have been applied to detect fraud patterns and anomalies in claims. These models help to identify potentially suspicious claims for further investigation. In 2018, for example, the system flagged 6,500 suspicious claims from 3.4 million claims, leading to quicker and more targeted reviews.

(iii) **Improved Accuracy and Speed:** The introduction of ML reduced the number of manual inspections, with claims that pass the automated checks being processed more efficiently. This speeds up payment processing and improves accuracy by catching errors earlier in the workflow.

(iv)  **Blockchain Technology for Data Security:** Estonia uses KSI Blockchain technology to ensure that patient and health care provider data are kept secure, reducing the risk of internal data breaches and ensuring the integrity of sensitive health records.

## Key Features and Benefits

The digital invoicing system and ML integration have led to significant improvements in the overall health care claims process in Estonia:

(i)   **Real-Time Claims Processing:** Providers can now submit claims in real time, reducing delays and administrative overhead. With immediate feedback on errors, providers can make necessary adjustments and resubmit claims quickly, ensuring accurate payments.

(ii)  **Fraud Prevention:** The ML models employed by the EHIF minimize the likelihood of fraudulent claims going undetected. The system ensures that no more than 5% of potentially fraudulent claims are missed, drastically improving fraud detection compared to traditional manual processes.

(iii) **Efficiency Gains:** Automated processes have greatly reduced the administrative workload for both the EHIF and health care providers. Payment processing is now faster, allowing providers to receive reimbursements with minimal delay and improving overall operational efficiency.

(iv)  **Cost Reduction:** Estonia's system has helped cut unnecessary health care costs by identifying and preventing fraudulent claims before payment. Moreover, reducing administrative overhead has saved time and resources, reducing overall expenses.

(v)   **Transparency and Compliance:** The EHIF provides transparency by publishing its claims verification controls online, allowing health care providers to adjust their systems to meet these requirements. This promotes a fair and consistent reimbursement process.

*continued on next page*

**Case Study 7** *continued*

## Impact

Adopting digital invoicing and ML has transformed Estonia's health care claims management system. The improvements are evident in both financial savings and operational efficiency:

(i)   **Enhanced Fraud Detection:** Before using ML, only a fraction of claims underwent scrutiny for fraud. With the new system in place, the number of claims requiring manual review has decreased, while the system ensures that fraudulent patterns are detected and flagged in real time.

(ii)  **Streamlined Operations for Providers:** Providers now benefit from automated contract monitoring, which compares real-time claims data with contract volumes, eliminating the need for extensive manual checks and interventions. This has allowed providers to manage their contract volumes more flexibly and transparently.

(iii) **Broader Health System Resilience:** The digitalization of Estonia's claims process has created a more resilient system capable of adapting to changing demands while ensuring financial sustainability. By using advanced digital tools, Estonia has managed to future-proof its health care financing system, making it more agile and responsive to potential economic downturns.

## Conclusion

Estonia's strategic implementation of digital invoicing and ML in health care has reduced FWA and enhanced its claims processing system's efficiency, transparency, and security. This case study highlights how a commitment to digital innovation can drive significant improvements in managing health care resources, ensuring sustainability and better outcomes for providers and patients.

Sources: Asian Development Bank. 2021. *Digital Technologies for Government-Supported Health Insurance Systems in Asia and the Pacific*; K. Kahur, et al. 2023. *The Role of Digital Claims Management for Estonia's Health Insurance.* Country Studies Series on Digital Technologies for Health Financing. World Health Organization; R. V. Jensen. 2020. *Digital Health Systems: A Comparison Between Estonia and New Zealand.* University of Wellington.

**Case Study 8**

## Predictive Analytics in the United States

### Overview

A large health insurance company in the United States implemented a predictive analytics system to detect and prevent fraudulent claims. The system uses big data technologies and machine learning algorithms to analyze patterns and identify anomalies in billing and claims submissions.

### Technology Involved

(i)   Machine Learning Models: Algorithms that detect patterns and outliers based on historical claims data.

(ii)  Data Mining Tools: Used to extract and scrutinize vast amounts of data from various sources, including claims and provider data.

(iii) Natural Language Processing: To interpret and analyze the free text in insurance claims and clinical notes.

### Implementation

(i)   The insurance provider integrated these technologies into their existing claims processing systems.

(ii)  Training was provided for claims reviewers and investigators on how to interpret model outputs and decide on follow-up actions.

### Outcome

(i)   The predictive analytics system identified high-risk claims that were flagged for further investigation.

(ii)  Within the first year of implementation, the system helped save tens of millions of dollars by preventing fraudulent claims from being paid out.

(iii) The system also helped identify collusion between providers and patients who submit fraudulent claims, significantly reducing the loss ratios.

### Challenges

(i)   False positives were initially a significant challenge, requiring ongoing algorithm adjustments.

(ii)  The integration required substantial upfront investment in technology and training.

Sources: K. Weintraub. 2024. *Harnessing AI to Combat Fraud, Waste, and Abuse in Health Insurance.* Insurance Newsnet; Reward and Employee Benefits Association (REBA). 2018. *How to Tackle Health Insurance Fraud, Waste and Abuse: Everyone Has a Role to Play;* Ropes and Grey. 2024. 2024 U.S. Health Care Fraud, Waste and Abuse Trends (Part II): Guidance on Clinical Laboratory Arrangements.

## Case Study 9

# Detecting Prescription Fraud in the United Kingdom's National Health Service System

### Overview

The National Health Service (NHS) provides residents with medical care and prescriptions at subsidized rates or free of charge, making it a target for various types of fraud, waste, and abuse. Prescription fraud—obtaining or using prescriptions illegally to acquire medicines—can cost the NHS significant amounts annually. A specific instance involved the detection of high-risk prescriptions in a regional area where prescription volumes suddenly spiked unusually. Advanced machine learning algorithms analyzed these prescriptions and cross-referenced them with patient records and doctor orders. The system flagged these as potential fraud cases for further investigation.

### Objective

The objective was to implement an advanced analytics approach to identify, prevent, and manage prescription fraud, thus reducing associated costs and ensuring resources are used effectively.

### Implementation

#### Step 1: Data Collection

The NHS collected data from multiple sources, including pharmacies, general practitioners (GPs), and hospitals. The data encompassed patient records, prescription details, and dispensing information.

#### Step 2: Analytics Deployment

The NHS employed several advanced analytics techniques:

(i)   Predictive analytics were trained to forecast potentially fraudulent prescriptions based on historical fraud patterns.

(ii)   Machine learning models were trained on datasets of known fraudulent and legitimate prescriptions to identify characteristics of fraud.

(iii)   Text analytics were used to analyze the notes from GPs and other medical staff for discrepancies in prescription orders.

(iv)   Anomaly detection tools were used to identify outliers in prescription volumes or frequencies that did not correlate with diagnosed conditions.

#### Step 3: Real-Time Monitoring

Real-time data streaming and analysis were established, allowing the NHS to flag suspicious activities as prescriptions were processed. This system provided alerts whenever a prescription matched the characteristics of known fraud scenarios.

*continued on next page*

**Case Study 9** *continued*

## Investigation and actions taken

(i)   A dedicated NHS fraud prevention unit investigated the flagged cases. They discovered a scheme where specific individuals were forging prescriptions to obtain medications in bulk and selling them on the black market.

(ii)  The individuals involved were prosecuted, leading to convictions and recovery of substantial amounts of money. The doctors whose prescription pads were misused were also alerted, and additional security measures were implemented to improve their prescription processes.

## Results

(i)   **Cost Savings:** The prevention and recovery efforts saved the NHS millions of pounds in potential losses.

(ii)  **Improved Systems:** Enhanced detection systems deterred further fraudulent activities by increasing the risk of detection for fraudsters.

(iii) **Policy Changes:** The NHS updated its prescription policies, introducing more secure prescription forms and stricter pharmacy verification processes.

## Conclusion

Through the use of advanced analytics, the NHS was able to detect and manage prescription fraud effectively. This case study exemplifies how integrating technology into health care administration can significantly enhance the ability to safeguard resources, ensuring they are used for legitimate patient care. This proactive approach reduced the incidence of fraud and supported the overall integrity and efficiency of the health care system.

Sources: NHS Counter Fraud Authority. 2024. Strategic Intelligence Assessment 2024; National Health Service England. 2024. *Annual Report and Accounts 2023/24*; Government of the United Kingdom (UK), Department of Health and Social Care. 2024. Pharmacists Who Illegally Supplied More than 55 million Doses of Controlled Drugs Sentenced; York Health Economics Consortium. 2010. Evaluation of the Scale, Causes and Costs of Waste Medicines; NHS Business Services Authority. 2024. Fraud, Error and Loss Strategy 2024–2027; Government of the UK, Department of Health and Social Care. 2023. Stopping Fraud Against the NHS: New Plans Announced.

## Case Study 10

# The Republic of Korea National Health Insurance Service and the Use of Artificial Intelligence and Blockchain to Combat Fraud, Waste, and Abuse

### Overview

The Republic of Korea's National Health Insurance Service (NHIS) manages the country's universal health coverage, which serves over 51 million people. Like many health care systems, the NHIS faces ongoing challenges with fraud, waste, and abuse (FWA) in medical claims and service delivery. To address these issues, the NHIS has integrated artificial intelligence (AI), big data analytics, and, more recently, blockchain technology into its operations. These technologies aim to enhance fraud detection and improve the security and transparency of health care transactions.

### Application of Blockchain by the NHIS

The NHIS began piloting blockchain technology as part of its broader initiative to digitalize health care claims management and secure patient data. The NHIS specifically targeted the use of blockchain to improve the traceability and security of medical records and billing within the health care system. Blockchain's decentralized nature provides an immutable ledger that records and time-stamps every transaction related to health care claims and payments and is unalterable. This technology helps reduce FWA by ensuring that records cannot be tampered with or falsified.

The NHIS implements one specific blockchain in collaboration with the Health Insurance Review and Assessment Service (HIRA), which reviews and processes claims. The blockchain platform allows the NHIS and HIRA to verify the authenticity of claims in real time by cross-referencing patient data and service records from different providers on a secure, shared ledger. This significantly reduces the chances of fraudulent claims being submitted.

### Benefits of Blockchain Technology

(i)  **Enhanced Transparency and Traceability:** Blockchain ensures that every step in the claims process is recorded and visible to authorized parties, creating a transparent audit trail. This makes it easier for the NHIS and HIRA to detect irregularities or anomalies in claims submissions. For example, it can instantly detect any attempt to alter medical records or duplicate billing entries.

(ii)  **Improved Data Security:** With blockchain, patient records and billing data are encrypted and stored across multiple nodes, making it virtually impossible for hackers to alter or steal sensitive information. This reduces the risk of data breaches, historically a significant issue in health care systems worldwide. By securing data at every transaction point, the NHIS ensures that patient and financial data remains safe from cyber threats.

(iii)  **Streamlined Claims Processing:** Blockchain has helped streamline the claims process by reducing the need for intermediaries and manual verification steps. With a single, secure source of truth accessible to all parties involved, the NHIS can process claims more efficiently, reducing administrative overhead and speeding up provider reimbursements.

*continued on next page*

**Case Study 10** *continued*

## Risks and Challenges

(i) **Technological Integration:** One of the main challenges the NHIS faces is integrating blockchain technology into an existing health care infrastructure already heavily reliant on AI and big data analytics. Combining these technologies requires significant investment in system upgrades, staff training, and cybersecurity measures.

(ii) **Data Privacy and Regulatory Compliance:** While blockchain offers improved security, it raises questions about data privacy, especially concerning compliance with the Republic of Korea's strict data protection laws. The NHIS must ensure its blockchain system complies with the Personal Information Protection Act and other personal health data regulations.

(iii) **Scalability:** As the NHIS looks to scale its blockchain implementation across the entire health care system, there are concerns about its ability to handle a high volume of transactions. While secure, blockchain technology can sometimes suffer latency and scalability issues, particularly when large amounts of data are processed simultaneously.

## Conclusion

The introduction of blockchain technology by the NHIS represents a significant step forward in combating FWA in the Republic of Korea's health care system. By enhancing the transparency, security, and efficiency of claims processing, blockchain complements existing AI and data analytics tools, creating a robust defense against FWA. The NHIS must continue to address technological integration, data privacy, and scalability challenges to realize blockchain benefits fully.

Sources: International Social Security Association (ISSA). 2021. *Operation of Machine Learning-based Fraud Detection and Prediction System;* S. Chhabra, et al. 2018. Preventing, Detecting and Deterring Fraud in Social Health Insurance Programs: Lessons from Selected Countries. *Health, Nutrition and Population Discussion Paper.* World Bank.

**Case Study 11**

# Indonesia's Use of Technology to Address Fraud, Waste, and Abuse in Health Care

## Overview

Indonesia's National Health Insurance (Jaminan Kesehatan Nasional) program—managed by BPJS Kesehatan—is the world's largest single-payer health insurance system, covering more than 220 million Indonesians. However, the program faces fraud, waste, and abuse (FWA) challenges in health care claims. BPJS Kesehatan has implemented various technology-driven initiatives to combat these issues, including digital claims submission systems and data analytics tools to enhance fraud detection and prevention.

## Application of Technology

BPJS Kesehatan has adopted the e-Claim system, an electronic claims submission platform that allows healthcare providers to submit claims digitally. This system reduces manual errors and helps in the early detection of suspicious claims. It also enables the organization to track patterns and trends in healthcare service utilization, making it easier to spot anomalies that may indicate fraud, such as overcharging or unnecessary medical procedures.

BPJS Kesehatan uses big data analytics to process and analyze claims data. By comparing claims from different healthcare providers and regions, the system can detect inconsistencies in billing practices. For example, the system can flag healthcare providers who submit a higher-than-average number of claims for specific procedures, which may signal potential abuse.

## Benefits of Technology for Addressing FWA

(i)   **Increased Efficiency in Claims Processing:** The e-Claim system has greatly improved claims processing efficiency, reducing the time it takes to review and approve claims. By automating the process, BPJS Kesehatan can handle the large volume of claims it receives daily while minimizing the risk of errors and fraudulent claims slipping through the system.

(ii)  **Data-Driven Fraud Detection:** The use of big data analytics allows BPJS Kesehatan to identify patterns of fraudulent activity that would be difficult to detect manually. For example, the system can analyze the frequency of specific treatments or procedures across different providers and flag outliers for further investigation.

(iii) **Cost Savings:** BPJS Kesehatan has saved substantial money by reducing fraud and preventing the payout of fraudulent claims. These savings are crucial for the sustainability of Indonesia's universal healthcare system, which is under financial pressure due to the sheer size of the population it covers.

*continued on next page*

**Case Study 11** *continued*

## Challenges and Risks

(i) **Technological Infrastructure and Training:** While the e-Claim system and data analytics tools have improved efficiency, smaller healthcare providers, particularly in rural areas, may lack the technological infrastructure to integrate with these systems fully. Additionally, ongoing training for healthcare staff on using these tools is essential to ensure they are effectively implemented.

(ii) **Data Privacy and Security:** As with any system handling large volumes of sensitive patient data, there are risks associated with data privacy and security. BPJS Kesehatan must ensure the systems comply with Indonesia's data protection laws to prevent unauthorized access and data breaches.

(iii) **Evolving Nature of Fraud:** Fraudsters continually adapt their tactics to exploit weaknesses in the system. BPJS Kesehatan must regularly update its fraud detection algorithms and data analytics capabilities to stay ahead of new forms of abuse, which requires ongoing investment in technology.

## Conclusion

Indonesia's adoption of technology to combat FWA in its national health insurance system has significantly improved claims processing efficiency and fraud detection. Using digital claims platforms and data analytics has helped reduce financial losses due to fraud while also improving transparency and accountability in the healthcare system. Challenges related to technological infrastructure, data security, and evolving fraud tactics must be continuously addressed to ensure the long-term success of these initiatives.

Sources: W. H. Saputra, Agus Prima. 2022. E-Claim System for Health Insurance and Social Security (BPJS) Types in Indonesia: Innovation and Effectiveness of Services. *Journal of Society Medicine.* 1 (1); Asrori and Y. Hikmah. 2018. Analysis of Health Insurance Claim Decisions in Indonesia. *Advances in Social Science, Education and Humanities Research,* Vol. 426. 3rd International Conference on Vocational Higher Education (ICVHE); D. S. Susanti, et al. 2022. *Tackling Fraud and Corruption in Indonesia's Health Insurance System.* U4 Anti-Corruption Resource Centre; N. Munaa, et al. 2020. *Fraud Detection in Indonesia National Health Insurance Implementation: A Phenomenology Experience from Hospital.* International Conference of Business and Social Sciences.

## Case Study 12

# Addressing Fraud in Health Insurance Operations in the Philippines

### Overview

The Philippine Health Insurance Corporation (PhilHealth) is crucial for providing health insurance coverage for millions of Filipinos. However, like many health systems globally, it faces significant challenges with fraud, waste, and abuse (FWA). PhilHealth has turned to digital platforms, fraud detection algorithms, and a centralized claims processing system to address fraudulent claims and inefficiencies.

### Application of Technology

PhilHealth's efforts to combat FWA focus on integrating technology in claims processing and monitoring. One of the major initiatives is the development of the PhilHealth Claims Processing Information System, a digital platform that standardizes and automates the evaluation of claims submitted by healthcare providers. This system incorporates rules and algorithms designed to flag suspicious claims and identify inconsistencies, such as patterns of overcharging or the submission of duplicate claims.

PhilHealth is exploring using artificial intelligence (AI) and data analytics to enhance fraud detection capabilities. These systems allow real-time data analysis and help identify fraud patterns across multiple healthcare providers. By leveraging AI, PhilHealth can focus its investigations on high-risk claims, reducing the likelihood of paying out fraudulent or inflated claims.

### Benefits of Technology for Addressing FWA

(i)   **Improved Detection and Prevention:** Through digital claims processing and AI-powered analysis, PhilHealth has significantly improved its ability to detect fraudulent activities. This has led to a more efficient claims review process, reducing the time and resources required to identify potential fraud cases. The ability to analyze large amounts of claims data in real time ensures that high-risk claims are flagged before payments are made.

(ii)  **Transparency and Accountability:** The centralized claims processing system enhances transparency in the billing and reimbursement processes. By having a digital record of all transactions, it is easier to track patterns of abuse, hold providers accountable, and reduce incidents of overbilling. This system also reduces opportunities for manual tampering, thus increasing the integrity of the claims review process.

(iii) **Cost Savings and Efficiency:** By reducing fraudulent claims, PhilHealth can allocate resources more efficiently, directing funds toward genuine healthcare needs. The reduction in fraud directly translates into lower operating costs for the payer, which ultimately helps sustain the insurance pool for more members.

*continued on next page*

**Case Study 12** *continued*

## Challenges and Risks

(i) **Technological Infrastructure and Integration:** While the digital claims processing system is a step forward, there are challenges related to technology integration across a fragmented healthcare landscape in the Philippines. Not all healthcare providers have the technological capacity or knowledge to fully utilize digital systems, which can create inefficiencies and gaps in fraud detection.

(ii) **Data Privacy and Security:** With the introduction of AI and extensive data collection, PhilHealth must ensure strict compliance with the Philippines' Data Privacy Act. Safeguarding sensitive patient data is crucial, and any breaches could lead to legal consequences, loss of public trust, and further financial losses.

(iii) **Evolving Nature of Fraud:** Fraud schemes are constantly evolving, and fraudsters often find new ways to exploit gaps in the system. While AI and technology can help reduce fraud, continuous updates to the algorithms and systems are necessary to avoid new types of fraud, such as falsified medical records or inflated claims for unnecessary procedures.

## Conclusion

PhilHealth's use of digital technology and AI has significantly enhanced its ability to combat FWA in the Philippines' healthcare system. Integrating a centralized claims processing system, combined with data analytics and AI, has improved fraud detection and increased transparency and accountability within the system. Challenges related to infrastructure, data privacy, and the evolving nature of fraud continue to pose risks. Despite these challenges, the technological innovations being implemented by PhilHealth represent a crucial step toward a more efficient and transparent healthcare system.

Sources: Development Academy of the Philippines, Center of Excellence on Public Sector Productivity (COE-PSP). 2024. *PhilHealth Region V Integrity Drive: A Data Analytics Solution for Healthcare Fraud Detection and Prevention.* 24 June; Philippine Health Insurance Corporation (PhilHealth). 2019. *PhilHealth Adopts State-of-the-Art Technology to Fight Fraud.* 6 November; M. Oranje and I. Mathauer. 2024. Exploring the Effects of Digital Technologies in Health Financing for Universal Health Coverage: A Synthesis of Country Experiences and Lessons. *Oxford Open Digital Health*, Vol. 2; A. Ulitin, et al. 2022. Measuring the Extent of Fraudulent-Risky Benefit Claims in PhilHealth Development of a Fraud Risk Index for PhilHealth Benefit Claims. *Science and Engineering Journal.* 15 (Supplement). pp. 34–42. October.

# CONCLUSIONS



Addressing FWA represents one of the most significant opportunities for health care payers. It offers the opportunity to make substantial cost savings to ensure long-term scheme viability, sustain universal health coverage gains, and identify practices that could otherwise lead to suboptimal clinical outcomes. But health care payers need to act swiftly. While providing a vital suite of solutions to support FWA management, technology has allowed new and increasingly sophisticated FWA schemes to emerge. Though perhaps unwilling participants, health care payers are increasingly racing to keep one step ahead and impact people's lives.

# APPENDIX

## Overview of Survey Participant Profiles

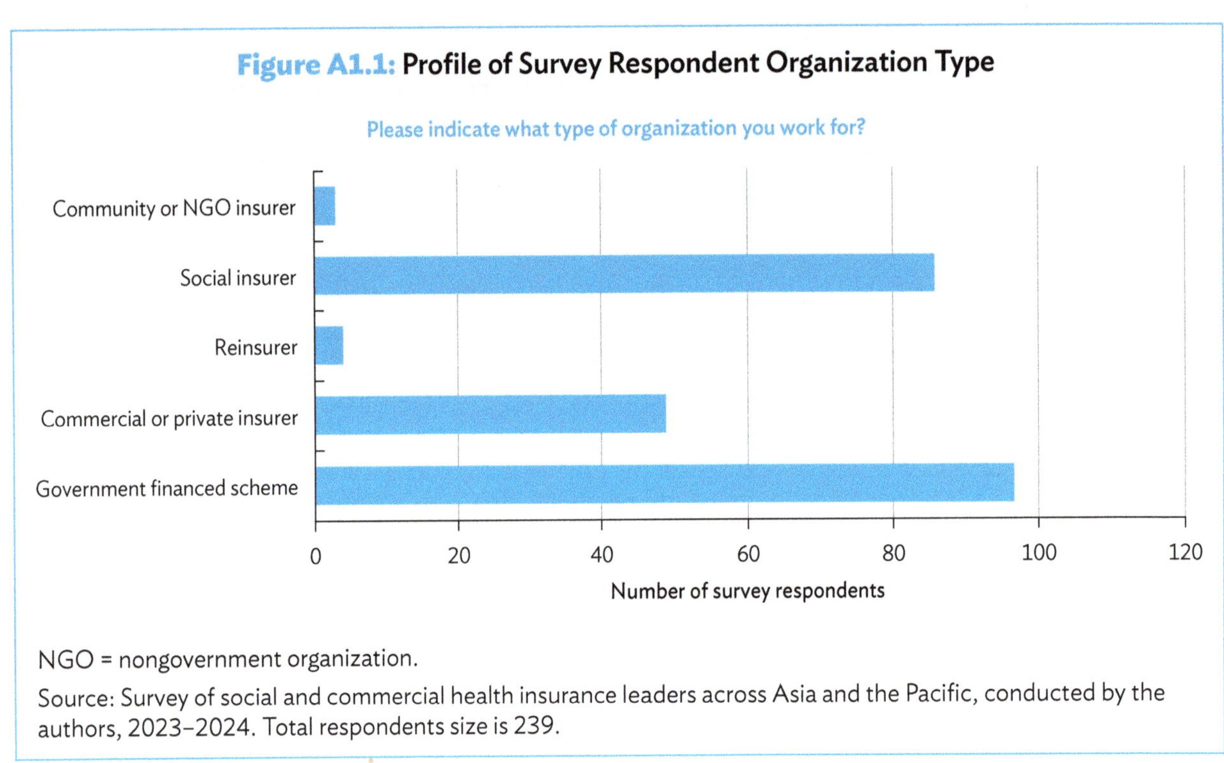



NGO = nongovernment organization.

Source: Survey of social and commercial health insurance leaders across Asia and the Pacific, conducted by the authors, 2023–2024. Total respondents size is 239.

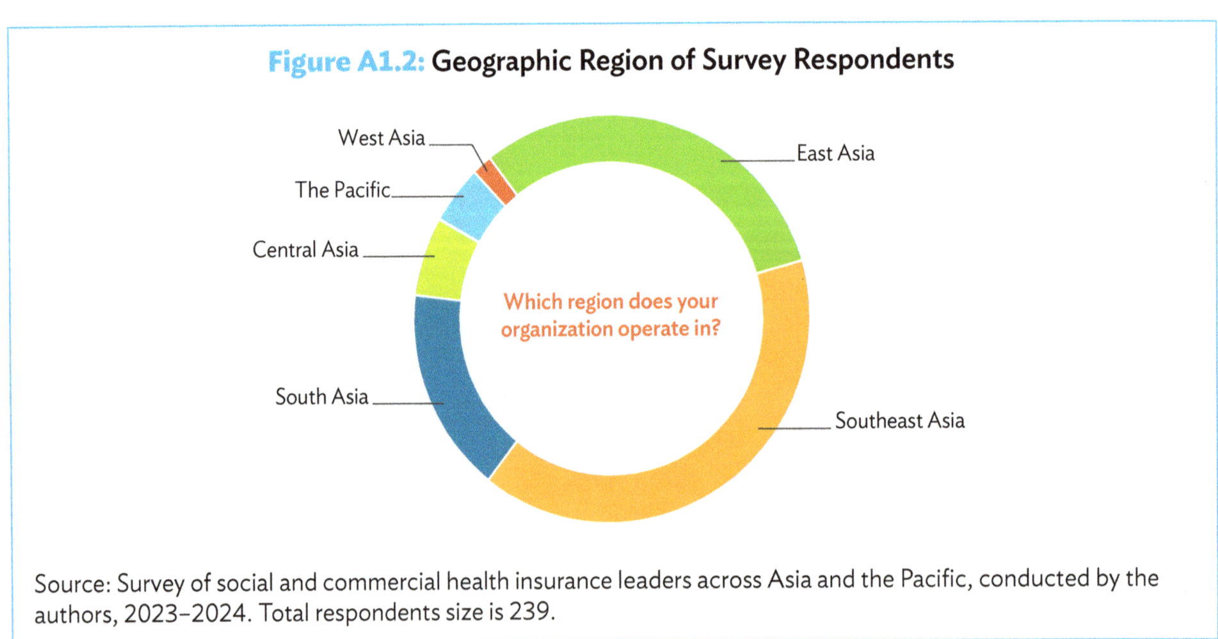



Source: Survey of social and commercial health insurance leaders across Asia and the Pacific, conducted by the authors, 2023–2024. Total respondents size is 239.

# REFERENCES

Frontiers in Public Health. 2021. How Do Moral Hazard Behaviors Lead to the Waste of Medical Insurance Funds? An Empirical Study from China.

Hong, B. et al. 2024. Health Insurance Fraud Detection Based on Multi-Channel Heterogeneous Graph Structure Learning. *Heliyon.* 10 (9). 24 April.

Mackey, T. K. and B. A. Liang. 2012. Combating Healthcare Corruption and Fraud with Improved Global Health Governance. *BMC International Health and Human Rights.* 12 (1). p. 23.

Nabrawi, E. and A. Alanazi. 2023. Fraud Detection in Healthcare Insurance Claims Using Machine Learning. *Risks.* 11 (9). p. 160. MDPI.

Organisation for Economic Co-operation and Development (OECD). 2017. Tackling Wasteful Spending on Health. 10 January.

———. 2020. Health at a Glance 2020: OECD Indicators (accessed 1 July 2024).

———. 2021. *Preventing Corruption: Public Procurement.*

Stiernstedt, P. and G. Brooks. 2020. Preventing Fraud and Providing Services: The Private Healthcare Insurance Sector. *Security Journal.* 34. pp. 621–634.

United Nations Development Programme. 2011. *Fighting Corruption in the Health Sector: Methods, Tools, and Good Practices.*

United Nations Office on Drugs and Crime. 2004. *The Global Programme against Corruption: UN Anti-Corruption Toolkit.*

Weintraub, K. 2024. Harnessing AI to combat fraud, waste, and abuse in health insurance. Insurance Newsnet.

World Health Organization (WHO). 2010. *The World Health Report 2010—Health Systems Financing: The Path to Universal Coverage.*

———. 2019. *Global Spending on Health: A World in Transition.*

———. 2021. *Digital Technologies for Health Financing: What Are the Benefits and Risks for UHC?*

———. 2021. *SCORE for Health Data Technical Package: Global Report on Health Data Systems and Capacity, 2020.*